W0374334

INTERNATIONAL HEALTH REGULATIONS (2005)

SECOND EDITION

INTERNATIONAL HEALTH REGULATIONS (2005)

SECOND EDITION

World Health Organization

WHO Library Cataloguing-in-Publication Data

International health regulations (2005) -- 2nd ed.

1. Legislation, Health. 2. Communicable disease control - legislation. 3. Disease notification - legislation. 4. International cooperation. I.World Health Organization. II.Title: IHR (2005).

ISBN 978 92 4 158041 0 (NLM classification: WA 32.1)

Printed in Switzerland

CONTENTS

INTERNATIONAL HEALTH REGULATIONS (2005)

ANNEXES

APPENDICES

FOREWORD

A central and historic responsibility for the World Health Organization (WHO) has been the management of the global regime for the control of the international spread of disease. Under Articles 21(a) and 22, the Constitution of WHO confers upon the World Health Assembly the authority to adopt regulations "designed to prevent the international spread of disease" which, after adoption by the Health Assembly, enter into force for all WHO Member States that do not affirmatively opt out of them within a specified time period.

The International Health Regulations ("the IHR" or "Regulations") were adopted by the Health Assembly in 1969[1], having been preceded by the International Sanitary Regulations adopted by the Fourth World Health Assembly in 1951. The 1969 Regulations, which initially covered six "quarantinable diseases" were amended in 1973[2] and 1981[3], primarily to reduce the number of covered diseases from six to three (yellow fever, plague and cholera) and to mark the global eradication of smallpox.

In consideration of the growth in international travel and trade, and the emergence or re-emergence of international disease threats and other public health risks, the Forty-eighth World Health Assembly in 1995 called for a substantial revision of the Regulations adopted in 1969[4]. In resolution WHA48.7, the Health Assembly requested the Director-General to take steps to prepare their revision, urging broad participation and cooperation in the process.

After extensive preliminary work on the revision by WHO's Secretariat in close consultation with WHO Member States, international organizations and other relevant partners, and the momentum created by the emergence of severe acute respiratory syndrome (the first global public health emergency of the 21st century)[5], the Health Assembly established an Intergovernmental Working Group in 2003 open to all Member States to review and recommend a draft revision of the Regulations to the Health Assembly[6]. The IHR (2005) were adopted by the Fifty-eighth World Health Assembly on 23 May 2005[7]. They entered into force on 15 June 2007.

The purpose and scope of the IHR (2005) are "to prevent, protect against, control and provide a public health response to the international spread of disease in ways that are commensurate with and restricted to public health risks, and which avoid unnecessary interference with international traffic and trade." The IHR (2005) contain a range of innovations, including: (a) a scope not limited to any specific disease or manner of transmission, but covering "illness or medical condition, irrespective of origin or source, that presents or could present significant harm to humans"; (b) State Party obligations to develop certain minimum core public health capacities; (c) obligations on States Parties to notify WHO of events that may constitute a public health emergency of international concern according to defined criteria; (d) provisions authorizing WHO to take into consideration unofficial reports of public health events and to obtain verification from States Parties concerning such events; (e) procedures for the determination by the Director-General of a "public health emergency of international concern" and issuance of corresponding temporary recommendations, after taking into account the views of an Emergency Committee; (f) protection of the human rights of persons and travellers; and (g) the

[1] See WHO Official Records, No. 176, 1969, resolution WHA22.46 and Annex I.
[2] See WHO Official Records, No. 209, 1973, resolution WHA26.55.
[3] See document WHA34/1981/REC/1 resolution WHA34.13; see also WHO Official Records, No. 217, 1974, resolution WHA27.45, and resolution EB67.R13, Amendment of the International Health Regulations (1969).
[4] See resolution WHA48.7.
[5] See resolution WHA56.29.
[6] See resolution WHA56.28.
[7] See resolution WHA58.3.

establishment of National IHR Focal Points and WHO IHR Contact Points for urgent communications between States Parties and WHO.

By not limiting the application of the IHR (2005) to specific diseases, it is intended that the Regulations will maintain their relevance and applicability for many years to come even in the face of the continued evolution of diseases and of the factors determining their emergence and transmission. The provisions in the IHR (2005) also update and revise many of the technical and other regulatory functions, including certificates applicable to international travel and transport, and requirements for international ports, airports and ground crossings.

This second edition contains the text of the IHR (2005), the text of World Health Assembly resolution WHA58.3, the version of the Health Part of the Aircraft General Declaration that entered into force on 15 July 2007, appendices containing a list of States Parties and State Party reservations and other communications in connection with the IHR (2005).

REVISION OF THE INTERNATIONAL HEALTH REGULATIONS

The Fifty-eighth World Health Assembly,

Having considered the draft revised International Health Regulations[1];

Having regard to articles 2(*k*), 21(*a*) and 22 of the Constitution of WHO;

Recalling references to the need for revising and updating the International Health Regulations in resolutions WHA48.7 on revision and updating of the International Health Regulations, WHA54.14 on global health security: epidemic alert and response, WHA55.16 on global public health response to natural occurrence, accidental release or deliberate use of biological and chemical agents or radionuclear material that affect health, WHA56.28 on revision of the International Health Regulations, and WHA56.29 on severe acute respiratory syndrome (SARS), with a view to responding to the need to ensure global public health;

Welcoming resolution 58/3 of the United Nations General Assembly on enhancing capacity building in global public health, which underscores the importance of the International Health Regulations and urges that high priority should be given to their revision;

Affirming the continuing importance of WHO's role in global outbreak alert and response to public health events, in accordance with its mandate;

Underscoring the continued importance of the International Health Regulations as the key global instrument for protection against the international spread of disease;

Commending the successful conclusion of the work of the Intergovernmental Working Group on Revision of the International Health Regulations,

1. ADOPTS the revised International Health Regulations attached to this resolution, to be referred to as the "International Health Regulations (2005)";

2. CALLS UPON Member States and the Director-General to implement fully the International Health Regulations (2005), in accordance with the purpose and scope set out in Article 2 and the principles embodied in Article 3;

3. DECIDES, for the purposes of paragraph 1 of Article 54 of the International Health Regulations (2005), that States Parties and the Director-General shall submit their first report to the Sixty-first World Health Assembly, and that the Health Assembly shall on that occasion consider the schedule for the submission of further such reports and the first review on the functioning of the Regulations pursuant to paragraph 2 of Article 54;

4. FURTHER DECIDES that, for the purposes of paragraph 1 of Article 14 of the International Health Regulations (2005), the other competent intergovernmental organizations or international bodies with which WHO is expected to cooperate and coordinate its activities, as appropriate, include the following: United Nations, International Labour Organization, Food and Agriculture Organization, International Atomic Energy Agency, International Civil Aviation Organization, International Maritime Organization, International Committee of the Red Cross, International Federation of Red

---

[1] See document A58/4.

Cross and Red Crescent Societies, International Air Transport Association, International Shipping Federation, and *Office International des Epizooties*;

5. URGES Member States:

(1) to build, strengthen and maintain the capacities required under the International Health Regulations (2005), and to mobilize the resources necessary for that purpose;

(2) to collaborate actively with each other and WHO in accordance with the relevant provisions of the International Health Regulations (2005), so as to ensure their effective implementation;

(3) to provide support to developing countries and countries with economies in transition if they so request in the building, strengthening and maintenance of the public health capacities required under the International Health Regulations (2005);

(4) to take all appropriate measures for furthering the purpose and eventual implementation of the International Health Regulations (2005) pending their entry into force, including development of the necessary public health capacities and legal and administrative provisions, and, in particular, to initiate the process for introducing use of the decision instrument contained in Annex 2;

6. REQUESTS the Director-General:

(1) to give prompt notification of adoption of the International Health Regulations (2005) in accordance with paragraph 1 of Article 65 thereof;

(2) to inform other competent intergovernmental organizations or international bodies of adoption of the International Health Regulations (2005) and, as appropriate, to cooperate with them in the updating of their norms and standards and to coordinate with them the activities of WHO under the International Health Regulations (2005) with a view to ensuring application of adequate measures for the protection of public health and strengthening of the global public-health response to the international spread of disease;

(3) to transmit to the International Civil Aviation Organization (ICAO) the recommended changes to the Health Part of the Aircraft General Declaration,[1] and, after completion by ICAO of its revision of the Aircraft General Declaration, to inform the Health Assembly and replace Annex 9 of the International Health Regulations (2005) with the Health Part of the Aircraft General Declaration as revised by ICAO;

(4) to build and strengthen the capacities of WHO to perform fully and effectively the functions entrusted to it under the International Health Regulations (2005), in particular through strategic health operations that provide support to countries in detection and assessment of, and response to, public health emergencies;

(5) to collaborate with States Parties to the International Health Regulations (2005), as appropriate, including through the provision or facilitation of technical cooperation and logistical support;

(6) to collaborate with States Parties to the extent possible in the mobilization of financial resources to provide support to developing countries in building, strengthening and maintaining the capacities required under the International Health Regulations (2005);

---

[1] Document A58/41 Add.2.

(7) to draw up, in consultation with Member States, guidelines for the application of health measures at ground crossings in accordance with Article 29 of the International Health Regulations (2005);

(8) to establish the Review Committee of the International Health Regulations (2005) in accordance with Article 50 of the Regulations;

(9) to take steps immediately to prepare guidelines for implementation and evaluation of the decision instrument contained in the International Health Regulations (2005), including elaboration of a procedure for review of its functioning, which shall be submitted to the Health Assembly for its consideration pursuant to paragraph 3 of Article 54 of the Regulations;

(10) to take steps to establish an IHR Roster of Experts and to invite proposals for its membership, pursuant to Article 47 of the International Health Regulations (2005).

INTERNATIONAL HEALTH REGULATIONS (2005)

PART I – DEFINITIONS, PURPOSE AND SCOPE, PRINCIPLES AND RESPONSIBLE AUTHORITIES

Article 1 Definitions

1. For the purposes of the International Health Regulations (hereinafter "the IHR" or "Regulations"):

"affected" means persons, baggage, cargo, containers, conveyances, goods, postal parcels or human remains that are infected or contaminated, or carry sources of infection or contamination, so as to constitute a public health risk;

"affected area" means a geographical location specifically for which health measures have been recommended by WHO under these Regulations;

"aircraft" means an aircraft making an international voyage;

"airport" means any airport where international flights arrive or depart;

"arrival" of a conveyance means:

(a) in the case of a seagoing vessel, arrival or anchoring in the defined area of a port;

(b) in the case of an aircraft, arrival at an airport;

(c) in the case of an inland navigation vessel on an international voyage, arrival at a point of entry;

(d) in the case of a train or road vehicle, arrival at a point of entry;

"baggage" means the personal effects of a traveller;

"cargo" means goods carried on a conveyance or in a container;

"competent authority" means an authority responsible for the implementation and application of health measures under these Regulations;

"container" means an article of transport equipment:

(a) of a permanent character and accordingly strong enough to be suitable for repeated use;

(b) specially designed to facilitate the carriage of goods by one or more modes of transport, without intermediate reloading;

(c) fitted with devices permitting its ready handling, particularly its transfer from one mode of transport to another; and

(d) specially designed as to be easy to fill and empty;

"container loading area" means a place or facility set aside for containers used in international traffic;

"contamination" means the presence of an infectious or toxic agent or matter on a human or animal body surface, in or on a product prepared for consumption or on other inanimate objects, including conveyances, that may constitute a public health risk;

"conveyance" means an aircraft, ship, train, road vehicle or other means of transport on an international voyage;

"conveyance operator" means a natural or legal person in charge of a conveyance or their agent;

"crew" means persons on board a conveyance who are not passengers;

"decontamination" means a procedure whereby health measures are taken to eliminate an infectious or toxic agent or matter on a human or animal body surface, in or on a product prepared for consumption or on other inanimate objects, including conveyances, that may constitute a public health risk;

"departure" means, for persons, baggage, cargo, conveyances or goods, the act of leaving a territory;

"deratting" means the procedure whereby health measures are taken to control or kill rodent vectors of human disease present in baggage, cargo, containers, conveyances, facilities, goods and postal parcels at the point of entry;

"Director-General" means the Director-General of the World Health Organization;

"disease" means an illness or medical condition, irrespective of origin or source, that presents or could present significant harm to humans;

"disinfection" means the procedure whereby health measures are taken to control or kill infectious agents on a human or animal body surface or in or on baggage, cargo, containers, conveyances, goods and postal parcels by direct exposure to chemical or physical agents;

"disinsection" means the procedure whereby health measures are taken to control or kill the insect vectors of human diseases present in baggage, cargo, containers, conveyances, goods and postal parcels;

"event" means a manifestation of disease or an occurrence that creates a potential for disease;

"*free pratique*" means permission for a ship to enter a port, embark or disembark, discharge or load cargo or stores; permission for an aircraft, after landing, to embark or disembark, discharge or load cargo or stores; and permission for a ground transport vehicle, upon arrival, to embark or disembark, discharge or load cargo or stores;

"goods" mean tangible products, including animals and plants, transported on an international voyage, including for utilization on board a conveyance;

"ground crossing" means a point of land entry in a State Party, including one utilized by road vehicles and trains;

"ground transport vehicle" means a motorized conveyance for overland transport on an international voyage, including trains, coaches, lorries and automobiles;

"health measure" means procedures applied to prevent the spread of disease or contamination; a health measure does not include law enforcement or security measures;

"ill person" means an individual suffering from or affected with a physical ailment that may pose a public health risk;

"infection" means the entry and development or multiplication of an infectious agent in the body of humans and animals that may constitute a public health risk;

"inspection" means the examination, by the competent authority or under its supervision, of areas, baggage, containers, conveyances, facilities, goods or postal parcels, including relevant data and documentation, to determine if a public health risk exists;

"international traffic" means the movement of persons, baggage, cargo, containers, conveyances, goods or postal parcels across an international border, including international trade;

"international voyage" means:

(a) in the case of a conveyance, a voyage between points of entry in the territories of more than one State, or a voyage between points of entry in the territory or territories of the same State if the conveyance has contacts with the territory of any other State on its voyage but only as regards those contacts;

(b) in the case of a traveller, a voyage involving entry into the territory of a State other than the territory of the State in which that traveller commences the voyage;

"intrusive" means possibly provoking discomfort through close or intimate contact or questioning;

"invasive" means the puncture or incision of the skin or insertion of an instrument or foreign material into the body or the examination of a body cavity. For the purposes of these Regulations, medical examination of the ear, nose and mouth, temperature assessment using an ear, oral or cutaneous thermometer, or thermal imaging; medical inspection; auscultation; external palpation; retinoscopy; external collection of urine, faeces or saliva samples; external measurement of blood pressure; and electrocardiography shall be considered to be non-invasive;

"isolation" means separation of ill or contaminated persons or affected baggage, containers, conveyances, goods or postal parcels from others in such a manner as to prevent the spread of infection or contamination;

"medical examination" means the preliminary assessment of a person by an authorized health worker or by a person under the direct supervision of the competent authority, to determine the person's health status and potential public health risk to others, and may include the scrutiny of health documents, and a physical examination when justified by the circumstances of the individual case;

"National IHR Focal Point" means the national centre, designated by each State Party, which shall be accessible at all times for communications with WHO IHR Contact Points under these Regulations;

"Organization" or "WHO" means the World Health Organization;

"permanent residence" has the meaning as determined in the national law of the State Party concerned;

"personal data" means any information relating to an identified or identifiable natural person;

"point of entry" means a passage for international entry or exit of travellers, baggage, cargo, containers, conveyances, goods and postal parcels as well as agencies and areas providing services to them on entry or exit;

"port" means a seaport or a port on an inland body of water where ships on an international voyage arrive or depart;

"postal parcel" means an addressed article or package carried internationally by postal or courier services;

"public health emergency of international concern" means an extraordinary event which is determined, as provided in these Regulations:

(i) to constitute a public health risk to other States through the international spread of disease and

(ii) to potentially require a coordinated international response;

"public health observation" means the monitoring of the health status of a traveller over time for the purpose of determining the risk of disease transmission;

"public health risk" means a likelihood of an event that may affect adversely the health of human populations, with an emphasis on one which may spread internationally or may present a serious and direct danger;

"quarantine" means the restriction of activities and/or separation from others of suspect persons who are not ill or of suspect baggage, containers, conveyances or goods in such a manner as to prevent the possible spread of infection or contamination;

"recommendation" and "recommended" refer to temporary or standing recommendations issued under these Regulations;

"reservoir" means an animal, plant or substance in which an infectious agent normally lives and whose presence may constitute a public health risk;

"road vehicle" means a ground transport vehicle other than a train;

"scientific evidence" means information furnishing a level of proof based on the established and accepted methods of science;

"scientific principles" means the accepted fundamental laws and facts of nature known through the methods of science;

"ship" means a seagoing or inland navigation vessel on an international voyage;

"standing recommendation" means non-binding advice issued by WHO for specific ongoing public health risks pursuant to Article 16 regarding appropriate health measures for routine or periodic application needed to prevent or reduce the international spread of disease and minimize interference with international traffic;

"surveillance" means the systematic ongoing collection, collation and analysis of data for public health purposes and the timely dissemination of public health information for assessment and public health response as necessary;

"suspect" means those persons, baggage, cargo, containers, conveyances, goods or postal parcels considered by a State Party as having been exposed, or possibly exposed, to a public health risk and that could be a possible source of spread of disease;

"temporary recommendation" means non-binding advice issued by WHO pursuant to Article 15 for application on a time-limited, risk-specific basis, in response to a public health emergency of international concern, so as to prevent or reduce the international spread of disease and minimize interference with international traffic;

"temporary residence" has the meaning as determined in the national law of the State Party concerned;

"traveller" means a natural person undertaking an international voyage;

"vector" means an insect or other animal which normally transports an infectious agent that constitutes a public health risk;

"verification" means the provision of information by a State Party to WHO confirming the status of an event within the territory or territories of that State Party;

"WHO IHR Contact Point" means the unit within WHO which shall be accessible at all times for communications with the National IHR Focal Point.

2. Unless otherwise specified or determined by the context, reference to these Regulations includes the annexes thereto.

Article 2 Purpose and scope

The purpose and scope of these Regulations are to prevent, protect against, control and provide a public health response to the international spread of disease in ways that are commensurate with and restricted to public health risks, and which avoid unnecessary interference with international traffic and trade.

Article 3 Principles

1. The implementation of these Regulations shall be with full respect for the dignity, human rights and fundamental freedoms of persons.

2. The implementation of these Regulations shall be guided by the Charter of the United Nations and the Constitution of the World Health Organization.

3. The implementation of these Regulations shall be guided by the goal of their universal application for the protection of all people of the world from the international spread of disease.

4. States have, in accordance with the Charter of the United Nations and the principles of international law, the sovereign right to legislate and to implement legislation in pursuance of their health policies. In doing so they should uphold the purpose of these Regulations.

Article 4 Responsible authorities

1. Each State Party shall designate or establish a National IHR Focal Point and the authorities responsible within its respective jurisdiction for the implementation of health measures under these Regulations.

2. National IHR Focal Points shall be accessible at all times for communications with the WHO IHR Contact Points provided for in paragraph 3 of this Article. The functions of National IHR Focal Points shall include:

(a) sending to WHO IHR Contact Points, on behalf of the State Party concerned, urgent communications concerning the implementation of these Regulations, in particular under Articles 6 to 12; and

(b) disseminating information to, and consolidating input from relevant sectors of the administration of the State Party concerned, including those responsible for surveillance and reporting, points of entry, public health services, clinics and hospitals and other government departments.

3. WHO shall designate IHR Contact Points, which shall be accessible at all times for communications with National IHR Focal Points. WHO IHR Contact Points shall send urgent communications concerning the implementation of these Regulations, in particular under Articles 6 to 12, to the National IHR Focal Point of the States Parties concerned. WHO IHR Contact Points may be designated by WHO at the headquarters or at the regional level of the Organization.

4. States Parties shall provide WHO with contact details of their National IHR Focal Point and WHO shall provide States Parties with contact details of WHO IHR Contact Points. These contact details shall be continuously updated and annually confirmed. WHO shall make available to all States Parties the contact details of National IHR Focal Points it receives pursuant to this Article.

PART II – INFORMATION AND PUBLIC HEALTH RESPONSE

Article 5 Surveillance

1. Each State Party shall develop, strengthen and maintain, as soon as possible but no later than five years from the entry into force of these Regulations for that State Party, the capacity to detect, assess, notify and report events in accordance with these Regulations, as specified in Annex 1.

2. Following the assessment referred to in paragraph 2, Part A of Annex 1, a State Party may report to WHO on the basis of a justified need and an implementation plan and, in so doing, obtain an extension of two years in which to fulfil the obligation in paragraph 1 of this Article. In exceptional circumstances, and supported by a new implementation plan, the State Party may request a further extension not exceeding two years from the Director-General, who shall make the decision, taking into account the technical advice of the Committee established under Article 50 (hereinafter the "Review Committee"). After the period mentioned in paragraph 1 of this Article, the State Party that has obtained an extension shall report annually to WHO on progress made towards the full implementation.

3. WHO shall assist States Parties, upon request, to develop, strengthen and maintain the capacities referred to in paragraph 1 of this Article.

4. WHO shall collect information regarding events through its surveillance activities and assess their potential to cause international disease spread and possible interference with international traffic. Information received by WHO under this paragraph shall be handled in accordance with Articles 11 and 45 where appropriate.

Article 6 Notification

1. Each State Party shall assess events occurring within its territory by using the decision instrument in Annex 2. Each State Party shall notify WHO, by the most efficient means of communication available, by way of the National IHR Focal Point, and within 24 hours of assessment of public health information, of all events which may constitute a public health emergency of international concern within its territory in accordance with the decision instrument, as well as any health measure implemented in response to those events. If the notification received by WHO involves the competency of the International Atomic Energy Agency (IAEA), WHO shall immediately notify the IAEA.

2. Following a notification, a State Party shall continue to communicate to WHO timely, accurate and sufficiently detailed public health information available to it on the notified event, where possible including case definitions, laboratory results, source and type of the risk, number of cases and deaths, conditions affecting the spread of the disease and the health measures employed; and report, when necessary, the difficulties faced and support needed in responding to the potential public health emergency of international concern.

Article 7 Information-sharing during unexpected or unusual public health events

If a State Party has evidence of an unexpected or unusual public health event within its territory, irrespective of origin or source, which may constitute a public health emergency of international concern, it shall provide to WHO all relevant public health information. In such a case, the provisions of Article 6 shall apply in full.

Article 8 Consultation

In the case of events occurring within its territory not requiring notification as provided in Article 6, in particular those events for which there is insufficient information available to complete the decision instrument, a State Party may nevertheless keep WHO advised thereof through the National IHR Focal Point and consult with WHO on appropriate health measures. Such communications shall be treated in accordance with paragraphs 2 to 4 of Article 11. The State Party in whose territory the event has occurred may request WHO assistance to assess any epidemiological evidence obtained by that State Party.

Article 9 Other reports

1. WHO may take into account reports from sources other than notifications or consultations and shall assess these reports according to established epidemiological principles and then communicate information on the event to the State Party in whose territory the event is allegedly occurring. Before taking any action based on such reports, WHO shall consult with and attempt to obtain verification from the State Party in whose territory the event is allegedly occurring in accordance with the procedure set forth in Article 10. To this end, WHO shall make the information received available to the States Parties and only where it is duly justified may WHO maintain the confidentiality of the source. This information will be used in accordance with the procedure set forth in Article 11.

2. States Parties shall, as far as practicable, inform WHO within 24 hours of receipt of evidence of a public health risk identified outside their territory that may cause international disease spread, as manifested by exported or imported:

(a) human cases;

(b) vectors which carry infection or contamination; or

(c) goods that are contaminated.

Article 10 Verification

1. WHO shall request, in accordance with Article 9, verification from a State Party of reports from sources other than notifications or consultations of events which may constitute a public health emergency of international concern allegedly occurring in the State's territory. In such cases, WHO shall inform the State Party concerned regarding the reports it is seeking to verify.

2. Pursuant to the foregoing paragraph and to Article 9, each State Party, when requested by WHO, shall verify and provide:

(a) within 24 hours, an initial reply to, or acknowledgement of, the request from WHO;

(b) within 24 hours, available public health information on the status of events referred to in WHO's request; and

(c) information to WHO in the context of an assessment under Article 6, including relevant information as described in that Article.

3. When WHO receives information of an event that may constitute a public health emergency of international concern, it shall offer to collaborate with the State Party concerned in assessing the potential for international disease spread, possible interference with international traffic and the adequacy of control measures. Such activities may include collaboration with other standard-setting organizations and the offer to mobilize international assistance in order to support the national authorities in conducting and coordinating on-site assessments. When requested by the State Party, WHO shall provide information supporting such an offer.

4. If the State Party does not accept the offer of collaboration, WHO may, when justified by the magnitude of the public health risk, share with other States Parties the information available to it, whilst encouraging the State Party to accept the offer of collaboration by WHO, taking into account the views of the State Party concerned.

Article 11 Provision of information by WHO

1. Subject to paragraph 2 of this Article, WHO shall send to all States Parties and, as appropriate, to relevant intergovernmental organizations, as soon as possible and by the most efficient means available, in confidence, such public health information which it has received under Articles 5 to 10 inclusive and which is necessary to enable States Parties to respond to a public health risk. WHO should communicate information to other States Parties that might help them in preventing the occurrence of similar incidents.

2. WHO shall use information received under Articles 6 and 8 and paragraph 2 of Article 9 for verification, assessment and assistance purposes under these Regulations and, unless otherwise agreed with the States Parties referred to in those provisions, shall not make this information generally available to other States Parties, until such time as:

(a) the event is determined to constitute a public health emergency of international concern in accordance with Article 12; or

(b) information evidencing the international spread of the infection or contamination has been confirmed by WHO in accordance with established epidemiological principles; or

(c) there is evidence that:

(i) control measures against the international spread are unlikely to succeed because of the nature of the contamination, disease agent, vector or reservoir; or

(ii) the State Party lacks sufficient operational capacity to carry out necessary measures to prevent further spread of disease; or

(d) the nature and scope of the international movement of travellers, baggage, cargo, containers, conveyances, goods or postal parcels that may be affected by the infection or contamination requires the immediate application of international control measures.

3. WHO shall consult with the State Party in whose territory the event is occurring as to its intent to make information available under this Article.

4. When information received by WHO under paragraph 2 of this Article is made available to States Parties in accordance with these Regulations, WHO may also make it available to the public if other information about the same event has already become publicly available and there is a need for the dissemination of authoritative and independent information.

Article 12 Determination of a public health emergency of international concern

1. The Director-General shall determine, on the basis of the information received, in particular from the State Party within whose territory an event is occurring, whether an event constitutes a public health emergency of international concern in accordance with the criteria and the procedure set out in these Regulations.

2. If the Director-General considers, based on an assessment under these Regulations, that a public health emergency of international concern is occurring, the Director-General shall consult with the State Party in whose territory the event arises regarding this preliminary determination. If the Director-General and the State Party are in agreement regarding this determination, the Director-General shall, in accordance with the procedure set forth in Article 49, seek the views of the Committee established under Article 48 (hereinafter the "Emergency Committee") on appropriate temporary recommendations.

3. If, following the consultation in paragraph 2 above, the Director-General and the State Party in whose territory the event arises do not come to a consensus within 48 hours on whether the event constitutes a public health emergency of international concern, a determination shall be made in accordance with the procedure set forth in Article 49.

4. In determining whether an event constitutes a public health emergency of international concern, the Director-General shall consider:

(a) information provided by the State Party;

(b) the decision instrument contained in Annex 2;

(c) the advice of the Emergency Committee;

(d) scientific principles as well as the available scientific evidence and other relevant information; and

(e) an assessment of the risk to human health, of the risk of international spread of disease and of the risk of interference with international traffic.

5. If the Director-General, following consultations with the State Party within whose territory the public health emergency of international concern has occurred, considers that a public health emergency of international concern has ended, the Director-General shall take a decision in accordance with the procedure set out in Article 49.

Article 13 Public health response

1. Each State Party shall develop, strengthen and maintain, as soon as possible but no later than five years from the entry into force of these Regulations for that State Party, the capacity to respond promptly and effectively to public health risks and public health emergencies of international concern as set out in Annex 1. WHO shall publish, in consultation with Member States, guidelines to support States Parties in the development of public health response capacities.

2. Following the assessment referred to in paragraph 2, Part A of Annex 1, a State Party may report to WHO on the basis of a justified need and an implementation plan and, in so doing, obtain an extension of two years in which to fulfil the obligation in paragraph 1 of this Article. In exceptional circumstances and supported by a new implementation plan, the State Party may request a further extension not exceeding two years from the Director-General, who shall make the decision, taking into account the technical advice of the Review Committee. After the period mentioned in paragraph 1 of this Article, the State Party that has obtained an extension shall report annually to WHO on progress made towards the full implementation.

3. At the request of a State Party, WHO shall collaborate in the response to public health risks and other events by providing technical guidance and assistance and by assessing the effectiveness of the control measures in place, including the mobilization of international teams of experts for on-site assistance, when necessary.

4. If WHO, in consultation with the States Parties concerned as provided in Article 12, determines that a public health emergency of international concern is occurring, it may offer, in addition to the support indicated in paragraph 3 of this Article, further assistance to the State Party, including an assessment of the severity of the international risk and the adequacy of control measures. Such collaboration may include the offer to mobilize international assistance in order to support the national authorities in conducting and coordinating on-site assessments. When requested by the State Party, WHO shall provide information supporting such an offer.

5. When requested by WHO, States Parties should provide, to the extent possible, support to WHO-coordinated response activities.

6. When requested, WHO shall provide appropriate guidance and assistance to other States Parties affected or threatened by the public health emergency of international concern.

Article 14 Cooperation of WHO with intergovernmental organizations and international bodies

1. WHO shall cooperate and coordinate its activities, as appropriate, with other competent intergovernmental organizations or international bodies in the implementation of these Regulations, including through the conclusion of agreements and other similar arrangements.

2. In cases in which notification or verification of, or response to, an event is primarily within the competence of other intergovernmental organizations or international bodies, WHO shall coordinate its activities with such organizations or bodies in order to ensure the application of adequate measures for the protection of public health.

3. Notwithstanding the foregoing, nothing in these Regulations shall preclude or limit the provision by WHO of advice, support, or technical or other assistance for public health purposes.

PART III – RECOMMENDATIONS

Article 15 Temporary recommendations

1. If it has been determined in accordance with Article 12 that a public health emergency of international concern is occurring, the Director-General shall issue temporary recommendations in accordance with the procedure set out in Article 49. Such temporary recommendations may be modified or extended as appropriate, including after it has been determined that a public health emergency of international concern has ended, at which time other temporary recommendations may be issued as necessary for the purpose of preventing or promptly detecting its recurrence.

2. Temporary recommendations may include health measures to be implemented by the State Party experiencing the public health emergency of international concern, or by other States Parties, regarding persons, baggage, cargo, containers, conveyances, goods and/or postal parcels to prevent or reduce the international spread of disease and avoid unnecessary interference with international traffic.

3. Temporary recommendations may be terminated in accordance with the procedure set out in Article 49 at any time and shall automatically expire three months after their issuance. They may be modified or extended for additional periods of up to three months. Temporary recommendations may not continue beyond the second World Health Assembly after the determination of the public health emergency of international concern to which they relate.

Article 16 Standing recommendations

WHO may make standing recommendations of appropriate health measures in accordance with Article 53 for routine or periodic application. Such measures may be applied by States Parties regarding persons, baggage, cargo, containers, conveyances, goods and/or postal parcels for specific, ongoing public health risks in order to prevent or reduce the international spread of disease and avoid unnecessary interference with international traffic. WHO may, in accordance with Article 53, modify or terminate such recommendations, as appropriate.

Article 17 Criteria for recommendations

When issuing, modifying or terminating temporary or standing recommendations, the Director-General shall consider:

(a) the views of the States Parties directly concerned;

(b) the advice of the Emergency Committee or the Review Committee, as the case may be;

(c) scientific principles as well as available scientific evidence and information;

(d) health measures that, on the basis of a risk assessment appropriate to the circumstances, are not more restrictive of international traffic and trade and are not more intrusive to persons than reasonably available alternatives that would achieve the appropriate level of health protection;

(e) relevant international standards and instruments;

(f) activities undertaken by other relevant intergovernmental organizations and international bodies; and

(g) other appropriate and specific information relevant to the event.

With respect to temporary recommendations, the consideration by the Director-General of subparagraphs (e) and (f) of this Article may be subject to limitations imposed by urgent circumstances.

Article 18 Recommendations with respect to persons, baggage, cargo, containers, conveyances, goods and postal parcels

1. Recommendations issued by WHO to States Parties with respect to persons may include the following advice:

- no specific health measures are advised;
- review travel history in affected areas;
- review proof of medical examination and any laboratory analysis;
- require medical examinations;
- review proof of vaccination or other prophylaxis;
- require vaccination or other prophylaxis;
- place suspect persons under public health observation;
- implement quarantine or other health measures for suspect persons;
- implement isolation and treatment where necessary of affected persons;
- implement tracing of contacts of suspect or affected persons;
- refuse entry of suspect and affected persons;
- refuse entry of unaffected persons to affected areas; and
- implement exit screening and/or restrictions on persons from affected areas.

2. Recommendations issued by WHO to States Parties with respect to baggage, cargo, containers, conveyances, goods and postal parcels may include the following advice:

- no specific health measures are advised;
- review manifest and routing;
- implement inspections;
- review proof of measures taken on departure or in transit to eliminate infection or contamination;
- implement treatment of the baggage, cargo, containers, conveyances, goods, postal parcels or human remains to remove infection or contamination, including vectors and reservoirs;
- the use of specific health measures to ensure the safe handling and transport of human remains;
- implement isolation or quarantine;

– seizure and destruction of infected or contaminated or suspect baggage, cargo, containers, conveyances, goods or postal parcels under controlled conditions if no available treatment or process will otherwise be successful; and

– refuse departure or entry.

PART IV – POINTS OF ENTRY

Article 19 General obligations

Each State Party shall, in addition to the other obligations provided for under these Regulations:

(a) ensure that the capacities set forth in Annex 1 for designated points of entry are developed within the timeframe provided in paragraph 1 of Article 5 and paragraph 1 of Article 13;

(b) identify the competent authorities at each designated point of entry in its territory; and

(c) furnish to WHO, as far as practicable, when requested in response to a specific potential public health risk, relevant data concerning sources of infection or contamination, including vectors and reservoirs, at its points of entry, which could result in international disease spread.

Article 20 Airports and ports

1. States Parties shall designate the airports and ports that shall develop the capacities provided in Annex 1.

2. States Parties shall ensure that Ship Sanitation Control Exemption Certificates and Ship Sanitation Control Certificates are issued in accordance with the requirements in Article 39 and the model provided in Annex 3.

3. Each State Party shall send to WHO a list of ports authorized to offer:

(a) the issuance of Ship Sanitation Control Certificates and the provision of the services referred to in Annexes 1 and 3; or

(b) the issuance of Ship Sanitation Control Exemption Certificates only; and

(c) extension of the Ship Sanitation Control Exemption Certificate for a period of one month until the arrival of the ship in the port at which the Certificate may be received.

Each State Party shall inform WHO of any changes which may occur to the status of the listed ports. WHO shall publish the information received under this paragraph.

4. WHO may, at the request of the State Party concerned, arrange to certify, after an appropriate investigation, that an airport or port in its territory meets the requirements referred to in paragraphs 1 and 3 of this Article. These certifications may be subject to periodic review by WHO, in consultation with the State Party.

5. WHO, in collaboration with competent intergovernmental organizations and international bodies, shall develop and publish the certification guidelines for airports and ports under this Article. WHO shall also publish a list of certified airports and ports.

Article 21 Ground crossings

1. Where justified for public health reasons, a State Party may designate ground crossings that shall develop the capacities provided in Annex 1, taking into consideration:

(a) the volume and frequency of the various types of international traffic, as compared to other points of entry, at a State Party's ground crossings which might be designated; and

(b) the public health risks existing in areas in which the international traffic originates, or through which it passes, prior to arrival at a particular ground crossing.

2. States Parties sharing common borders should consider:

(a) entering into bilateral or multilateral agreements or arrangements concerning prevention or control of international transmission of disease at ground crossings in accordance with Article 57; and

(b) joint designation of adjacent ground crossings for the capacities in Annex 1 in accordance with paragraph 1 of this Article.

Article 22 Role of competent authorities

1. The competent authorities shall:

(a) be responsible for monitoring baggage, cargo, containers, conveyances, goods, postal parcels and human remains departing and arriving from affected areas, so that they are maintained in such a condition that they are free of sources of infection or contamination, including vectors and reservoirs;

(b) ensure, as far as practicable, that facilities used by travellers at points of entry are maintained in a sanitary condition and are kept free of sources of infection or contamination, including vectors and reservoirs;

(c) be responsible for the supervision of any deratting, disinfection, disinsection or decontamination of baggage, cargo, containers, conveyances, goods, postal parcels and human remains or sanitary measures for persons, as appropriate under these Regulations;

(d) advise conveyance operators, as far in advance as possible, of their intent to apply control measures to a conveyance, and shall provide, where available, written information concerning the methods to be employed;

(e) be responsible for the supervision of the removal and safe disposal of any contaminated water or food, human or animal dejecta, wastewater and any other contaminated matter from a conveyance;

(f) take all practicable measures consistent with these Regulations to monitor and control the discharge by ships of sewage, refuse, ballast water and other potentially disease-causing matter which might contaminate the waters of a port, river, canal, strait, lake or other international waterway;

(g) be responsible for supervision of service providers for services concerning travellers, baggage, cargo, containers, conveyances, goods, postal parcels and human remains at points of entry, including the conduct of inspections and medical examinations as necessary;

(h) have effective contingency arrangements to deal with an unexpected public health event; and

(i) communicate with the National IHR Focal Point on the relevant public health measures taken pursuant to these Regulations.

2. Health measures recommended by WHO for travellers, baggage, cargo, containers, conveyances, goods, postal parcels and human remains arriving from an affected area may be reapplied on arrival, if there are verifiable indications and/or evidence that the measures applied on departure from the affected area were unsuccessful.

3. Disinsection, deratting, disinfection, decontamination and other sanitary procedures shall be carried out so as to avoid injury and as far as possible discomfort to persons, or damage to the environment in a way which impacts on public health, or damage to baggage, cargo, containers, conveyances, goods and postal parcels.

PART V – PUBLIC HEALTH MEASURES

Chapter I – General provisions

Article 23 Health measures on arrival and departure

1. Subject to applicable international agreements and relevant articles of these Regulations, a State Party may require for public health purposes, on arrival or departure:

(a) with regard to travellers:

(i) information concerning the traveller's destination so that the traveller may be contacted;

(ii) information concerning the traveller's itinerary to ascertain if there was any travel in or near an affected area or other possible contacts with infection or contamination prior to arrival, as well as review of the traveller's health documents if they are required under these Regulations; and/or

(iii) a non-invasive medical examination which is the least intrusive examination that would achieve the public health objective;

(b) inspection of baggage, cargo, containers, conveyances, goods, postal parcels and human remains.

2. On the basis of evidence of a public health risk obtained through the measures provided in paragraph 1 of this Article, or through other means, States Parties may apply additional health measures, in accordance with these Regulations, in particular, with regard to a suspect or affected traveller, on a case-by-case basis, the least intrusive and invasive medical examination that would achieve the public health objective of preventing the international spread of disease.

3. No medical examination, vaccination, prophylaxis or health measure under these Regulations shall be carried out on travellers without their prior express informed consent or that of their parents or guardians, except as provided in paragraph 2 of Article 31, and in accordance with the law and international obligations of the State Party.

4. Travellers to be vaccinated or offered prophylaxis pursuant to these Regulations, or their parents or guardians, shall be informed of any risk associated with vaccination or with non-vaccination and with the use or non-use of prophylaxis in accordance with the law and international obligations of the

State Party. States Parties shall inform medical practitioners of these requirements in accordance with the law of the State Party.

5. Any medical examination, medical procedure, vaccination or other prophylaxis which involves a risk of disease transmission shall only be performed on, or administered to, a traveller in accordance with established national or international safety guidelines and standards so as to minimize such a risk.

Chapter II – Special provisions for conveyances and conveyance operators

Article 24 Conveyance operators

1. States Parties shall take all practicable measures consistent with these Regulations to ensure that conveyance operators:

(a) comply with the health measures recommended by WHO and adopted by the State Party;

(b) inform travellers of the health measures recommended by WHO and adopted by the State Party for application on board; and

(c) permanently keep conveyances for which they are responsible free of sources of infection or contamination, including vectors and reservoirs. The application of measures to control sources of infection or contamination may be required if evidence is found.

2. Specific provisions pertaining to conveyances and conveyance operators under this Article are provided in Annex 4. Specific measures applicable to conveyances and conveyance operators with regard to vector-borne diseases are provided in Annex 5.

Article 25 Ships and aircraft in transit

Subject to Articles 27 and 43 or unless authorized by applicable international agreements, no health measure shall be applied by a State Party to:

(a) a ship not coming from an affected area which passes through a maritime canal or waterway in the territory of that State Party on its way to a port in the territory of another State. Any such ship shall be permitted to take on, under the supervision of the competent authority, fuel, water, food and supplies;

(b) a ship which passes through waters within its jurisdiction without calling at a port or on the coast; and

(c) an aircraft in transit at an airport within its jurisdiction, except that the aircraft may be restricted to a particular area of the airport with no embarking and disembarking or loading and discharging. However, any such aircraft shall be permitted to take on, under the supervision of the competent authority, fuel, water, food and supplies.

Article 26 Civilian lorries, trains and coaches in transit

Subject to Articles 27 and 43 or unless authorized by applicable international agreements, no health measure shall be applied to a civilian lorry, train or coach not coming from an affected area which passes through a territory without embarking, disembarking, loading or discharging.

Article 27 Affected conveyances

1. If clinical signs or symptoms and information based on fact or evidence of a public health risk, including sources of infection and contamination, are found on board a conveyance, the competent authority shall consider the conveyance as affected and may:

(a) disinfect, decontaminate, disinsect or derat the conveyance, as appropriate, or cause these measures to be carried out under its supervision; and

(b) decide in each case the technique employed to secure an adequate level of control of the public health risk as provided in these Regulations. Where there are methods or materials advised by WHO for these procedures, these should be employed, unless the competent authority determines that other methods are as safe and reliable.

The competent authority may implement additional health measures, including isolation of the conveyances, as necessary, to prevent the spread of disease. Such additional measures should be reported to the National IHR Focal Point.

2. If the competent authority for the point of entry is not able to carry out the control measures required under this Article, the affected conveyance may nevertheless be allowed to depart, subject to the following conditions:

(a) the competent authority shall, at the time of departure, inform the competent authority for the next known point of entry of the type of information referred to under subparagraph (b); and

(b) in the case of a ship, the evidence found and the control measures required shall be noted in the Ship Sanitation Control Certificate.

Any such conveyance shall be permitted to take on, under the supervision of the competent authority, fuel, water, food and supplies.

3. A conveyance that has been considered as affected shall cease to be regarded as such when the competent authority is satisfied that:

(a) the measures provided in paragraph 1 of this Article have been effectively carried out; and

(b) there are no conditions on board that could constitute a public health risk.

Article 28 Ships and aircraft at points of entry

1. Subject to Article 43 or as provided in applicable international agreements, a ship or an aircraft shall not be prevented for public health reasons from calling at any point of entry. However, if the point of entry is not equipped for applying health measures under these Regulations, the ship or aircraft may be ordered to proceed at its own risk to the nearest suitable point of entry available to it, unless the ship or aircraft has an operational problem which would make this diversion unsafe.

2. Subject to Article 43 or as provided in applicable international agreements, ships or aircraft shall not be refused *free pratique* by States Parties for public health reasons; in particular they shall not be prevented from embarking or disembarking, discharging or loading cargo or stores, or taking on fuel, water, food and supplies. States Parties may subject the granting of *free pratique* to inspection and, if a source of infection or contamination is found on board, the carrying out of necessary disinfection, decontamination, disinsection or deratting, or other measures necessary to prevent the spread of the infection or contamination.

3. Whenever practicable and subject to the previous paragraph, a State Party shall authorize the granting of *free pratique* by radio or other communication means to a ship or an aircraft when, on the basis of information received from it prior to its arrival, the State Party is of the opinion that the arrival of the ship or aircraft will not result in the introduction or spread of disease.

4. Officers in command of ships or pilots in command of aircraft, or their agents, shall make known to the port or airport control as early as possible before arrival at the port or airport of destination any cases of illness indicative of a disease of an infectious nature or evidence of a public health risk on board as soon as such illnesses or public health risks are made known to the officer or pilot. This information must be immediately relayed to the competent authority for the port or airport. In urgent circumstances, such information should be communicated directly by the officers or pilots to the relevant port or airport authority.

5. The following shall apply if a suspect or affected aircraft or ship, for reasons beyond the control of the pilot in command of the aircraft or the officer in command of the ship, lands elsewhere than at the airport at which the aircraft was due to land or berths elsewhere than at the port at which the ship was due to berth:

(a) the pilot in command of the aircraft or the officer in command of the ship or other person in charge shall make every effort to communicate without delay with the nearest competent authority;

(b) as soon as the competent authority has been informed of the landing it may apply health measures recommended by WHO or other health measures provided in these Regulations;

(c) unless required for emergency purposes or for communication with the competent authority, no traveller on board the aircraft or ship shall leave its vicinity and no cargo shall be removed from that vicinity, unless authorized by the competent authority; and

(d) when all health measures required by the competent authority have been completed, the aircraft or ship may, so far as such health measures are concerned, proceed either to the airport or port at which it was due to land or berth, or, if for technical reasons it cannot do so, to a conveniently situated airport or port.

6. Notwithstanding the provisions contained in this Article, the officer in command of a ship or pilot in command of an aircraft may take such emergency measures as may be necessary for the health and safety of travellers on board. He or she shall inform the competent authority as early as possible concerning any measures taken pursuant to this paragraph.

Article 29 Civilian lorries, trains and coaches at points of entry

WHO, in consultation with States Parties, shall develop guiding principles for applying health measures to civilian lorries, trains and coaches at points of entry and passing through ground crossings.

Chapter III – Special provisions for travellers

Article 30 Travellers under public health observation

Subject to Article 43 or as authorized in applicable international agreements, a suspect traveller who on arrival is placed under public health observation may continue an international voyage, if the traveller does not pose an imminent public health risk and the State Party informs the competent authority of the point of entry at destination, if known, of the traveller's expected arrival. On arrival, the traveller shall report to that authority.

Article 31 Health measures relating to entry of travellers

1. Invasive medical examination, vaccination or other prophylaxis shall not be required as a condition of entry of any traveller to the territory of a State Party, except that, subject to Articles 32, 42 and 45, these Regulations do not preclude States Parties from requiring medical examination, vaccination or other prophylaxis or proof of vaccination or other prophylaxis:

(a) when necessary to determine whether a public health risk exists;

(b) as a condition of entry for any travellers seeking temporary or permanent residence;

(c) as a condition of entry for any travellers pursuant to Article 43 or Annexes 6 and 7; or

(d) which may be carried out pursuant to Article 23.

2. If a traveller for whom a State Party may require a medical examination, vaccination or other prophylaxis under paragraph 1 of this Article fails to consent to any such measure, or refuses to provide the information or the documents referred to in paragraph 1(a) of Article 23, the State Party concerned may, subject to Articles 32, 42 and 45, deny entry to that traveller. If there is evidence of an imminent public health risk, the State Party may, in accordance with its national law and to the extent necessary to control such a risk, compel the traveller to undergo or advise the traveller, pursuant to paragraph 3 of Article 23, to undergo:

(a) the least invasive and intrusive medical examination that would achieve the public health objective;

(b) vaccination or other prophylaxis; or

(c) additional established health measures that prevent or control the spread of disease, including isolation, quarantine or placing the traveller under public health observation.

Article 32 Treatment of travellers

In implementing health measures under these Regulations, States Parties shall treat travellers with respect for their dignity, human rights and fundamental freedoms and minimize any discomfort or distress associated with such measures, including by:

(a) treating all travellers with courtesy and respect;

(b) taking into consideration the gender, sociocultural, ethnic or religious concerns of travellers; and

(c) providing or arranging for adequate food and water, appropriate accommodation and clothing, protection for baggage and other possessions, appropriate medical treatment, means of necessary communication if possible in a language that they can understand and other appropriate assistance for travellers who are quarantined, isolated or subject to medical examinations or other procedures for public health purposes.

Chapter IV – Special provisions for goods, containers and container loading areas

Article 33 Goods in transit

Subject to Article 43 or unless authorized by applicable international agreements, goods, other than live animals, in transit without transhipment shall not be subject to health measures under these Regulations or detained for public health purposes.

Article 34 Container and container loading areas

1. States Parties shall ensure, as far as practicable, that container shippers use international traffic containers that are kept free from sources of infection or contamination, including vectors and reservoirs, particularly during the course of packing.

2. States Parties shall ensure, as far as practicable, that container loading areas are kept free from sources of infection or contamination, including vectors and reservoirs.

3. Whenever, in the opinion of a State Party, the volume of international container traffic is sufficiently large, the competent authorities shall take all practicable measures consistent with these Regulations, including carrying out inspections, to assess the sanitary condition of container loading areas and containers in order to ensure that the obligations contained in these Regulations are implemented.

4. Facilities for the inspection and isolation of containers shall, as far as practicable, be available at container loading areas.

5. Container consignees and consignors shall make every effort to avoid cross-contamination when multiple-use loading of containers is employed.

PART VI – HEALTH DOCUMENTS

Article 35 General rule

No health documents, other than those provided for under these Regulations or in recommendations issued by WHO, shall be required in international traffic, provided however that this Article shall not apply to travellers seeking temporary or permanent residence, nor shall it apply to document requirements concerning the public health status of goods or cargo in international trade pursuant to applicable international agreements. The competent authority may request travellers to complete contact information forms and questionnaires on the health of travellers, provided that they meet the requirements set out in Article 23.

Article 36 Certificates of vaccination or other prophylaxis

1. Vaccines and prophylaxis for travellers administered pursuant to these Regulations, or to recommendations and certificates relating thereto, shall conform to the provisions of Annex 6 and, when applicable, Annex 7 with regard to specific diseases.

2. A traveller in possession of a certificate of vaccination or other prophylaxis issued in conformity with Annex 6 and, when applicable, Annex 7, shall not be denied entry as a consequence of the disease to which the certificate refers, even if coming from an affected area, unless the competent authority has verifiable indications and/or evidence that the vaccination or other prophylaxis was not effective.

Article 37 Maritime Declaration of Health

1. The master of a ship, before arrival at its first port of call in the territory of a State Party, shall ascertain the state of health on board, and, except when that State Party does not require it, the master shall, on arrival, or in advance of the vessel's arrival if the vessel is so equipped and the State Party requires such advance delivery, complete and deliver to the competent authority for that port a Maritime Declaration of Health which shall be countersigned by the ship's surgeon, if one is carried.

2. The master of a ship, or the ship's surgeon if one is carried, shall supply any information required by the competent authority as to health conditions on board during an international voyage.

3. A Maritime Declaration of Health shall conform to the model provided in Annex 8.

4. A State Party may decide:

(a) to dispense with the submission of the Maritime Declaration of Health by all arriving ships; or

(b) to require the submission of the Maritime Declaration of Health under a recommendation concerning ships arriving from affected areas or to require it from ships which might otherwise carry infection or contamination.

The State Party shall inform shipping operators or their agents of these requirements.

Article 38 Health Part of the Aircraft General Declaration

1. The pilot in command of an aircraft or the pilot's agent, in flight or upon landing at the first airport in the territory of a State Party, shall, to the best of his or her ability, except when that State Party does not require it, complete and deliver to the competent authority for that airport the Health Part of the Aircraft General Declaration which shall conform to the model specified in Annex 9.

2. The pilot in command of an aircraft or the pilot's agent shall supply any information required by the State Party as to health conditions on board during an international voyage and any health measure applied to the aircraft.

3. A State Party may decide:

(a) to dispense with the submission of the Health Part of the Aircraft General Declaration by all arriving aircraft; or

(b) to require the submission of the Health Part of the Aircraft General Declaration under a recommendation concerning aircraft arriving from affected areas or to require it from aircraft which might otherwise carry infection or contamination.

The State Party shall inform aircraft operators or their agents of these requirements.

Article 39 Ship sanitation certificates

1. Ship Sanitation Control Exemption Certificates and Ship Sanitation Control Certificates shall be valid for a maximum period of six months. This period may be extended by one month if the inspection or control measures required cannot be accomplished at the port.

2. If a valid Ship Sanitation Control Exemption Certificate or Ship Sanitation Control Certificate is not produced or evidence of a public health risk is found on board a ship, the State Party may proceed as provided in paragraph 1 of Article 27.

3. The certificates referred to in this Article shall conform to the model in Annex 3.

4. Whenever possible, control measures shall be carried out when the ship and holds are empty. In the case of a ship in ballast, they shall be carried out before loading.

5. When control measures are required and have been satisfactorily completed, the competent authority shall issue a Ship Sanitation Control Certificate, noting the evidence found and the control measures taken.

6. The competent authority may issue a Ship Sanitation Control Exemption Certificate at any port specified under Article 20 if it is satisfied that the ship is free of infection and contamination, including vectors and reservoirs. Such a certificate shall normally be issued only if the inspection of the ship has been carried out when the ship and holds are empty or when they contain only ballast or other material, of such a nature or so disposed as to make a thorough inspection of the holds possible.

7. If the conditions under which control measures are carried out are such that, in the opinion of the competent authority for the port where the operation was performed, a satisfactory result cannot be obtained, the competent authority shall make a note to that effect on the Ship Sanitation Control Certificate.

PART VII – CHARGES

Article 40 Charges for health measures regarding travellers

1. Except for travellers seeking temporary or permanent residence, and subject to paragraph 2 of this Article, no charge shall be made by a State Party pursuant to these Regulations for the following measures for the protection of public health:

(a) any medical examination provided for in these Regulations, or any supplementary examination which may be required by that State Party to ascertain the health status of the traveller examined;

(b) any vaccination or other prophylaxis provided to a traveller on arrival that is not a published requirement or is a requirement published less than 10 days prior to provision of the vaccination or other prophylaxis;

(c) appropriate isolation or quarantine requirements of travellers;

(d) any certificate issued to the traveller specifying the measures applied and the date of application; or

(e) any health measures applied to baggage accompanying the traveller.

2. States Parties may charge for health measures other than those referred to in paragraph 1 of this Article, including those primarily for the benefit of the traveller.

3. Where charges are made for applying such health measures to travellers under these Regulations, there shall be in each State Party only one tariff for such charges and every charge shall:

(a) conform to this tariff;

(b) not exceed the actual cost of the service rendered; and

(c) be levied without distinction as to the nationality, domicile or residence of the traveller concerned.

4. The tariff, and any amendment thereto, shall be published at least 10 days in advance of any levy thereunder.

5. Nothing in these Regulations shall preclude States Parties from seeking reimbursement for expenses incurred in providing the health measures in paragraph 1 of this Article:

(a) from conveyance operators or owners with regard to their employees; or

(b) from applicable insurance sources.

6. Under no circumstances shall travellers or conveyance operators be denied the ability to depart from the territory of a State Party pending payment of the charges referred to in paragraphs 1 or 2 of this Article.

Article 41 Charges for baggage, cargo, containers, conveyances, goods or postal parcels

1. Where charges are made for applying health measures to baggage, cargo, containers, conveyances, goods or postal parcels under these Regulations, there shall be in each State Party only one tariff for such charges and every charge shall:

(a) conform to this tariff;

(b) not exceed the actual cost of the service rendered; and

(c) be levied without distinction as to the nationality, flag, registry or ownership of the baggage, cargo, containers, conveyances, goods or postal parcels concerned. In particular, there shall be no distinction made between national and foreign baggage, cargo, containers, conveyances, goods or postal parcels.

2. The tariff, and any amendment thereto, shall be published at least 10 days in advance of any levy thereunder.

PART VIII – GENERAL PROVISIONS

Article 42 Implementation of health measures

Health measures taken pursuant to these Regulations shall be initiated and completed without delay, and applied in a transparent and non-discriminatory manner.

Article 43 Additional health measures

1. These Regulations shall not preclude States Parties from implementing health measures, in accordance with their relevant national law and obligations under international law, in response to specific public health risks or public health emergencies of international concern, which:

(a) achieve the same or greater level of health protection than WHO recommendations; or

(b) are otherwise prohibited under Article 25, Article 26, paragraphs 1 and 2 of Article 28, Article 30, paragraph 1(c) of Article 31 and Article 33,

provided such measures are otherwise consistent with these Regulations.

Such measures shall not be more restrictive of international traffic and not more invasive or intrusive to persons than reasonably available alternatives that would achieve the appropriate level of health protection.

2. In determining whether to implement the health measures referred to in paragraph 1 of this Article or additional health measures under paragraph 2 of Article 23, paragraph 1 of Article 27, paragraph 2 of Article 28 and paragraph 2(c) of Article 31, States Parties shall base their determinations upon:

(a) scientific principles;

(b) available scientific evidence of a risk to human health, or where such evidence is insufficient, the available information including from WHO and other relevant intergovernmental organizations and international bodies; and

(c) any available specific guidance or advice from WHO.

3. A State Party implementing additional health measures referred to in paragraph 1 of this Article which significantly interfere with international traffic shall provide to WHO the public health rationale and relevant scientific information for it. WHO shall share this information with other States Parties and shall share information regarding the health measures implemented. For the purpose of this Article, significant interference generally means refusal of entry or departure of international travellers, baggage, cargo, containers, conveyances, goods, and the like, or their delay, for more than 24 hours.

4. After assessing information provided pursuant to paragraph 3 and 5 of this Article and other relevant information, WHO may request that the State Party concerned reconsider the application of the measures.

5. A State Party implementing additional health measures referred to in paragraphs 1 and 2 of this Article that significantly interfere with international traffic shall inform WHO, within 48 hours of implementation, of such measures and their health rationale unless these are covered by a temporary or standing recommendation.

6. A State Party implementing a health measure pursuant to paragraph 1 or 2 of this Article shall within three months review such a measure taking into account the advice of WHO and the criteria in paragraph 2 of this Article.

7. Without prejudice to its rights under Article 56, any State Party impacted by a measure taken pursuant to paragraph 1 or 2 of this Article may request the State Party implementing such a measure to consult with it. The purpose of such consultations is to clarify the scientific information and public health rationale underlying the measure and to find a mutually acceptable solution.

8. The provisions of this Article may apply to implementation of measures concerning travellers taking part in mass congregations.

Article 44 Collaboration and assistance

1. States Parties shall undertake to collaborate with each other, to the extent possible, in:

(a) the detection and assessment of, and response to, events as provided under these Regulations;

(b) the provision or facilitation of technical cooperation and logistical support, particularly in the development, strengthening and maintenance of the public health capacities required under these Regulations;

(c) the mobilization of financial resources to facilitate implementation of their obligations under these Regulations; and

(d) the formulation of proposed laws and other legal and administrative provisions for the implementation of these Regulations.

2. WHO shall collaborate with States Parties, upon request, to the extent possible, in:

(a) the evaluation and assessment of their public health capacities in order to facilitate the effective implementation of these Regulations;

(b) the provision or facilitation of technical cooperation and logistical support to States Parties; and

(c) the mobilization of financial resources to support developing countries in building, strengthening and maintaining the capacities provided for in Annex 1.

3. Collaboration under this Article may be implemented through multiple channels, including bilaterally, through regional networks and the WHO regional offices, and through intergovernmental organizations and international bodies.

Article 45 Treatment of personal data

1. Health information collected or received by a State Party pursuant to these Regulations from another State Party or from WHO which refers to an identified or identifiable person shall be kept confidential and processed anonymously as required by national law.

2. Notwithstanding paragraph 1, States Parties may disclose and process personal data where essential for the purposes of assessing and managing a public health risk, but State Parties, in accordance with national law, and WHO must ensure that the personal data are:

(a) processed fairly and lawfully, and not further processed in a way incompatible with that purpose;

(b) adequate, relevant and not excessive in relation to that purpose;

(c) accurate and, where necessary, kept up to date; every reasonable step must be taken to ensure that data which are inaccurate or incomplete are erased or rectified; and

(d) not kept longer than necessary.

3. Upon request, WHO shall as far as practicable provide an individual with his or her personal data referred to in this Article in an intelligible form, without undue delay or expense and, when necessary, allow for correction.

Article 46 Transport and handling of biological substances, reagents and materials for diagnostic purposes

States Parties shall, subject to national law and taking into account relevant international guidelines, facilitate the transport, entry, exit, processing and disposal of biological substances and diagnostic specimens, reagents and other diagnostic materials for verification and public health response purposes under these Regulations.

PART IX – THE IHR ROSTER OF EXPERTS, THE EMERGENCY COMMITTEE AND THE REVIEW COMMITTEE

Chapter I – The IHR Roster of Experts

Article 47 Composition

The Director-General shall establish a roster composed of experts in all relevant fields of expertise (hereinafter the "IHR Expert Roster"). The Director-General shall appoint the members of the IHR Expert Roster in accordance with the WHO Regulations for Expert Advisory Panels and Committees (hereinafter the "WHO Advisory Panel Regulations"), unless otherwise provided in these Regulations. In addition, the Director-General shall appoint one member at the request of each State Party and, where appropriate, experts proposed by relevant intergovernmental and regional economic integration organizations. Interested States Parties shall notify the Director-General of the qualifications and fields of expertise of each of the experts they propose for membership. The Director-General shall periodically inform the States Parties, and relevant intergovernmental and regional economic integration organizations, of the composition of the IHR Expert Roster.

Chapter II – The Emergency Committee

Article 48 Terms of reference and composition

1. The Director-General shall establish an Emergency Committee that at the request of the Director-General shall provide its views on:

(a) whether an event constitutes a public health emergency of international concern;

(b) the termination of a public health emergency of international concern; and

(c) the proposed issuance, modification, extension or termination of temporary recommendations.

2. The Emergency Committee shall be composed of experts selected by the Director-General from the IHR Expert Roster and, when appropriate, other expert advisory panels of the Organization. The Director-General shall determine the duration of membership with a view to ensuring its continuity in the consideration of a specific event and its consequences. The Director-General shall select the members of the Emergency Committee on the basis of the expertise and experience required for any particular session and with due regard to the principles of equitable geographical representation. At least one member of the Emergency Committee should be an expert nominated by a State Party within whose territory the event arises.

3. The Director-General may, on his or her own initiative or at the request of the Emergency Committee, appoint one or more technical experts to advise the Committee.

Article 49 Procedure

1. The Director-General shall convene meetings of the Emergency Committee by selecting a number of experts from among those referred to in paragraph 2 of Article 48, according to the fields of expertise and experience most relevant to the specific event that is occurring. For the purpose of this Article, "meetings" of the Emergency Committee may include teleconferences, videoconferences or electronic communications.

2. The Director-General shall provide the Emergency Committee with the agenda and any relevant information concerning the event, including information provided by the States Parties, as well as any temporary recommendation that the Director-General proposes for issuance.

3. The Emergency Committee shall elect its Chairperson and prepare following each meeting a brief summary report of its proceedings and deliberations, including any advice on recommendations.

4. The Director-General shall invite the State Party in whose territory the event arises to present its views to the Emergency Committee. To that effect, the Director-General shall notify to it the dates and the agenda of the meeting of the Emergency Committee with as much advance notice as necessary. The State Party concerned, however, may not seek a postponement of the meeting of the Emergency Committee for the purpose of presenting its views thereto.

5. The views of the Emergency Committee shall be forwarded to the Director-General for consideration. The Director-General shall make the final determination on these matters.

6. The Director-General shall communicate to States Parties the determination and the termination of a public health emergency of international concern, any health measure taken by the State Party concerned, any temporary recommendation, and the modification, extension and termination of such recommendations, together with the views of the Emergency Committee. The Director-General shall inform conveyance operators through States Parties and the relevant international agencies of such temporary recommendations, including their modification, extension or termination. The Director-General shall subsequently make such information and recommendations available to the general public.

7. States Parties in whose territories the event has occurred may propose to the Director-General the termination of a public health emergency of international concern and/or the temporary recommendations, and may make a presentation to that effect to the Emergency Committee.

Chapter III – The Review Committee

Article 50 Terms of reference and composition

1. The Director-General shall establish a Review Committee, which shall carry out the following functions:

(a) make technical recommendations to the Director-General regarding amendments to these Regulations;

(b) provide technical advice to the Director-General with respect to standing recommendations, and any modifications or termination thereof;

(c) provide technical advice to the Director-General on any matter referred to it by the Director-General regarding the functioning of these Regulations.

2. The Review Committee shall be considered an expert committee and shall be subject to the WHO Advisory Panel Regulations, unless otherwise provided in this Article.

3. The Members of the Review Committee shall be selected and appointed by the Director-General from among the persons serving on the IHR Expert Roster and, when appropriate, other expert advisory panels of the Organization.

4. The Director-General shall establish the number of members to be invited to a meeting of the Review Committee, determine its date and duration, and convene the Committee.

5. The Director-General shall appoint members to the Review Committee for the duration of the work of a session only.

6. The Director-General shall select the members of the Review Committee on the basis of the principles of equitable geographical representation, gender balance, a balance of experts from developed and developing countries, representation of a diversity of scientific opinion, approaches and practical experience in various parts of the world, and an appropriate interdisciplinary balance.

Article 51 Conduct of business

1. Decisions of the Review Committee shall be taken by a majority of the members present and voting.

2. The Director-General shall invite Member States, the United Nations and its specialized agencies and other relevant intergovernmental organizations or nongovernmental organizations in official relations with WHO to designate representatives to attend the Committee sessions. Such representatives may submit memoranda and, with the consent of the Chairperson, make statements on the subjects under discussion. They shall not have the right to vote.

Article 52 Reports

1. For each session, the Review Committee shall draw up a report setting forth the Committee's views and advice. This report shall be approved by the Review Committee before the end of the session. Its views and advice shall not commit the Organization and shall be formulated as advice to the Director-General. The text of the report may not be modified without the Committee's consent.

2. If the Review Committee is not unanimous in its findings, any member shall be entitled to express his or her dissenting professional views in an individual or group report, which shall state the reasons why a divergent opinion is held and shall form part of the Committee's report.

3. The Review Committee's report shall be submitted to the Director-General, who shall communicate its views and advice to the Health Assembly or the Executive Board for their consideration and action.

Article 53 Procedures for standing recommendations

When the Director-General considers that a standing recommendation is necessary and appropriate for a specific public health risk, the Director-General shall seek the views of the Review Committee. In addition to the relevant paragraphs of Articles 50 to 52, the following provisions shall apply:

(a) proposals for standing recommendations, their modification or termination may be submitted to the Review Committee by the Director-General or by States Parties through the Director-General;

(b) any State Party may submit relevant information for consideration by the Review Committee;

(c) the Director-General may request any State Party, intergovernmental organization or nongovernmental organization in official relations with WHO to place at the disposal of the Review Committee information in its possession concerning the subject of the proposed standing recommendation as specified by the Review Committee;

(d) the Director-General may, at the request of the Review Committee or on the Director-General's own initiative, appoint one or more technical experts to advise the Review Committee. They shall not have the right to vote;

(e) any report containing the views and advice of the Review Committee regarding standing recommendations shall be forwarded to the Director-General for consideration and decision. The Director-General shall communicate the Review Committee's views and advice to the Health Assembly;

(f) the Director-General shall communicate to States Parties any standing recommendation, as well as the modifications or termination of such recommendations, together with the views of the Review Committee;

(g) standing recommendations shall be submitted by the Director-General to the subsequent Health Assembly for its consideration.

PART X – FINAL PROVISIONS

Article 54 Reporting and review

1. States Parties and the Director-General shall report to the Health Assembly on the implementation of these Regulations as decided by the Health Assembly.

2. The Health Assembly shall periodically review the functioning of these Regulations. To that end it may request the advice of the Review Committee, through the Director-General. The first such review shall take place no later than five years after the entry into force of these Regulations.

3. WHO shall periodically conduct studies to review and evaluate the functioning of Annex 2. The first such review shall commence no later than one year after the entry into force of these Regulations. The results of such reviews shall be submitted to the Health Assembly for its consideration, as appropriate.

Article 55 Amendments

1. Amendments to these Regulations may be proposed by any State Party or by the Director-General. Such proposals for amendments shall be submitted to the Health Assembly for its consideration.

2. The text of any proposed amendment shall be communicated to all States Parties by the Director-General at least four months before the Health Assembly at which it is proposed for consideration.

3. Amendments to these Regulations adopted by the Health Assembly pursuant to this Article shall come into force for all States Parties on the same terms, and subject to the same rights and obligations, as provided for in Article 22 of the Constitution of WHO and Articles 59 to 64 of these Regulations.

Article 56 Settlement of disputes

1. In the event of a dispute between two or more States Parties concerning the interpretation or application of these Regulations, the States Parties concerned shall seek in the first instance to settle

the dispute through negotiation or any other peaceful means of their own choice, including good offices, mediation or conciliation. Failure to reach agreement shall not absolve the parties to the dispute from the responsibility of continuing to seek to resolve it.

2. In the event that the dispute is not settled by the means described under paragraph 1 of this Article, the States Parties concerned may agree to refer the dispute to the Director-General, who shall make every effort to settle it.

3. A State Party may at any time declare in writing to the Director-General that it accepts arbitration as compulsory with regard to all disputes concerning the interpretation or application of these Regulations to which it is a party or with regard to a specific dispute in relation to any other State Party accepting the same obligation. The arbitration shall be conducted in accordance with the Permanent Court of Arbitration Optional Rules for Arbitrating Disputes between Two States applicable at the time a request for arbitration is made. The States Parties that have agreed to accept arbitration as compulsory shall accept the arbitral award as binding and final. The Director-General shall inform the Health Assembly regarding such action as appropriate.

4. Nothing in these Regulations shall impair the rights of States Parties under any international agreement to which they may be parties to resort to the dispute settlement mechanisms of other intergovernmental organizations or established under any international agreement.

5. In the event of a dispute between WHO and one or more States Parties concerning the interpretation or application of these Regulations, the matter shall be submitted to the Health Assembly.

Article 57 Relationship with other international agreements

1. States Parties recognize that the IHR and other relevant international agreements should be interpreted so as to be compatible. The provisions of the IHR shall not affect the rights and obligations of any State Party deriving from other international agreements.

2. Subject to paragraph 1 of this Article, nothing in these Regulations shall prevent States Parties having certain interests in common owing to their health, geographical, social or economic conditions, from concluding special treaties or arrangements in order to facilitate the application of these Regulations, and in particular with regard to:

(a) the direct and rapid exchange of public health information between neighbouring territories of different States;

(b) the health measures to be applied to international coastal traffic and to international traffic in waters within their jurisdiction;

(c) the health measures to be applied in contiguous territories of different States at their common frontier;

(d) arrangements for carrying affected persons or affected human remains by means of transport specially adapted for the purpose; and

(e) deratting, disinsection, disinfection, decontamination or other treatment designed to render goods free of disease-causing agents.

3. Without prejudice to their obligations under these Regulations, States Parties that are members of a regional economic integration organization shall apply in their mutual relations the common rules in force in that regional economic integration organization.

Article 58 International sanitary agreements and regulations

1. These Regulations, subject to the provisions of Article 62 and the exceptions hereinafter provided, shall replace as between the States bound by these Regulations and as between these States and WHO, the provisions of the following international sanitary agreements and regulations:

(a) International Sanitary Convention, signed in Paris, 21 June 1926;

(b) International Sanitary Convention for Aerial Navigation, signed at The Hague, 12 April 1933;

(c) International Agreement for dispensing with Bills of Health, signed in Paris, 22 December 1934;

(d) International Agreement for dispensing with Consular Visas on Bills of Health, signed in Paris, 22 December 1934;

(e) Convention modifying the International Sanitary Convention of 21 June 1926, signed in Paris, 31 October 1938;

(f) International Sanitary Convention, 1944, modifying the International Sanitary Convention of 21 June 1926, opened for signature in Washington, 15 December 1944;

(g) International Sanitary Convention for Aerial Navigation, 1944, modifying the International Sanitary Convention of 12 April 1933, opened for signature in Washington, 15 December 1944;

(h) Protocol of 23 April 1946 to prolong the International Sanitary Convention, 1944, signed in Washington;

(i) Protocol of 23 April 1946 to prolong the International Sanitary Convention for Aerial Navigation, 1944, signed in Washington;

(j) International Sanitary Regulations, 1951, and the Additional Regulations of 1955, 1956, 1960, 1963 and 1965; and

(k) the International Health Regulations of 1969 and the amendments of 1973 and 1981.

2. The Pan American Sanitary Code, signed at Havana, 14 November 1924, shall remain in force with the exception of Articles 2, 9, 10, 11, 16 to 53 inclusive, 61 and 62, to which the relevant part of paragraph 1 of this Article shall apply.

Article 59 Entry into force; period for rejection or reservations

1. The period provided in execution of Article 22 of the Constitution of WHO for rejection of, or reservation to, these Regulations or an amendment thereto, shall be 18 months from the date of the notification by the Director-General of the adoption of these Regulations or of an amendment to these Regulations by the Health Assembly. Any rejection or reservation received by the Director-General after the expiry of that period shall have no effect.

2. These Regulations shall enter into force 24 months after the date of notification referred to in paragraph 1 of this Article, except for:

(a) a State that has rejected these Regulations or an amendment thereto in accordance with Article 61;

(b) a State that has made a reservation, for which these Regulations shall enter into force as provided in Article 62;

(c) a State that becomes a Member of WHO after the date of the notification by the Director-General referred to in paragraph 1 of this Article, and which is not already a party to these Regulations, for which these Regulations shall enter into force as provided in Article 60; and

(d) a State not a Member of WHO that accepts these Regulations, for which they shall enter into force in accordance with paragraph 1 of Article 64.

3. If a State is not able to adjust its domestic legislative and administrative arrangements fully with these Regulations within the period set out in paragraph 2 of this Article, that State shall submit within the period specified in paragraph 1 of this Article a declaration to the Director-General regarding the outstanding adjustments and achieve them no later than 12 months after the entry into force of these Regulations for that State Party.

Article 60 New Member States of WHO

Any State which becomes a Member of WHO after the date of the notification by the Director-General referred to in paragraph 1 of Article 59, and which is not already a party to these Regulations, may communicate its rejection of, or any reservation to, these Regulations within a period of twelve months from the date of the notification to it by the Director-General after becoming a Member of WHO. Unless rejected, these Regulations shall enter into force with respect to that State, subject to the provisions of Articles 62 and 63, upon expiry of that period. In no case shall these Regulations enter into force in respect to that State earlier than 24 months after the date of notification referred to in paragraph 1 of Article 59.

Article 61 Rejection

If a State notifies the Director-General of its rejection of these Regulations or of an amendment thereto within the period provided in paragraph 1 of Article 59, these Regulations or the amendment concerned shall not enter into force with respect to that State. Any international sanitary agreement or regulations listed in Article 58 to which such State is already a party shall remain in force as far as such State is concerned.

Article 62 Reservations

1. States may make reservations to these Regulations in accordance with this Article. Such reservations shall not be incompatible with the object and purpose of these Regulations.

2. Reservations to these Regulations shall be notified to the Director-General in accordance with paragraph 1 of Article 59 and Article 60, paragraph 1 of Article 63 or paragraph 1 of Article 64, as the case may be. A State not a Member of WHO shall notify the Director-General of any reservation with its notification of acceptance of these Regulations. States formulating reservations should provide the Director-General with reasons for the reservations.

3. A rejection in part of these Regulations shall be considered as a reservation.

4. The Director-General shall, in accordance with paragraph 2 of Article 65, issue notification of each reservation received pursuant to paragraph 2 of this Article. The Director-General shall:

(a) if the reservation was made before the entry into force of these Regulations, request those Member States that have not rejected these Regulations to notify him or her within six months of any objection to the reservation, or

(b) if the reservation was made after the entry into force of these Regulations, request States Parties to notify him or her within six months of any objection to the reservation.

States objecting to a reservation should provide the Director-General with reasons for the objection.

5. After this period, the Director-General shall notify all States Parties of the objections he or she has received with regard to reservations. Unless by the end of six months from the date of the notification referred to in paragraph 4 of this Article a reservation has been objected to by one-third of the States referred to in paragraph 4 of this Article, it shall be deemed to be accepted and these Regulations shall enter into force for the reserving State, subject to the reservation.

6. If at least one-third of the States referred to in paragraph 4 of this Article object to the reservation by the end of six months from the date of the notification referred to in paragraph 4 of this Article, the Director-General shall notify the reserving State with a view to its considering withdrawing the reservation within three months from the date of the notification by the Director-General.

7. The reserving State shall continue to fulfil any obligations corresponding to the subject matter of the reservation, which the State has accepted under any of the international sanitary agreements or regulations listed in Article 58.

8. If the reserving State does not withdraw the reservation within three months from the date of the notification by the Director-General referred to in paragraph 6 of this Article, the Director-General shall seek the view of the Review Committee if the reserving State so requests. The Review Committee shall advise the Director-General as soon as possible and in accordance with Article 50 on the practical impact of the reservation on the operation of these Regulations.

9. The Director-General shall submit the reservation, and the views of the Review Committee if applicable, to the Health Assembly for its consideration. If the Health Assembly, by a majority vote, objects to the reservation on the ground that it is incompatible with the object and purpose of these Regulations, the reservation shall not be accepted and these Regulations shall enter into force for the reserving State only after it withdraws its reservation pursuant to Article 63. If the Health Assembly accepts the reservation, these Regulations shall enter into force for the reserving State, subject to its reservation.

Article 63 Withdrawal of rejection and reservation

1. A rejection made under Article 61 may at any time be withdrawn by a State by notifying the Director-General. In such cases, these Regulations shall enter into force with regard to that State upon receipt by the Director-General of the notification, except where the State makes a reservation when withdrawing its rejection, in which case these Regulations shall enter into force as provided in Article 62. In no case shall these Regulations enter into force in respect to that State earlier than 24 months after the date of notification referred to in paragraph 1 of Article 59.

2. The whole or part of any reservation may at any time be withdrawn by the State Party concerned by notifying the Director-General. In such cases, the withdrawal will be effective from the date of receipt by the Director-General of the notification.

Article 64 States not Members of WHO

1. Any State not a Member of WHO, which is a party to any international sanitary agreement or regulations listed in Article 58 or to which the Director-General has notified the adoption of these Regulations by the World Health Assembly, may become a party hereto by notifying its acceptance to the Director-General and, subject to the provisions of Article 62, such acceptance shall become effective upon the date of entry into force of these Regulations, or, if such acceptance is notified after that date, three months after the date of receipt by the Director-General of the notification of acceptance.

2. Any State not a Member of WHO which has become a party to these Regulations may at any time withdraw from participation in these Regulations, by means of a notification addressed to the Director-General which shall take effect six months after the Director-General has received it. The State which has withdrawn shall, as from that date, resume application of the provisions of any international sanitary agreement or regulations listed in Article 58 to which it was previously a party.

Article 65 Notifications by the Director-General

1. The Director-General shall notify all States Members and Associate Members of WHO, and also other parties to any international sanitary agreement or regulations listed in Article 58, of the adoption by the Health Assembly of these Regulations.

2. The Director-General shall also notify these States, as well as any other State which has become a party to these Regulations or to any amendment to these Regulations, of any notification received by WHO under Articles 60 to 64 respectively, as well as of any decision taken by the Health Assembly under Article 62.

Article 66 Authentic texts

1. The Arabic, Chinese, English, French, Russian and Spanish texts of these Regulations shall be equally authentic. The original texts of these Regulations shall be deposited with WHO.

2. The Director-General shall send, with the notification provided in paragraph 1 of Article 59, certified copies of these Regulations to all Members and Associate Members, and also to other parties to any of the international sanitary agreements or regulations listed in Article 58.

3. Upon the entry into force of these Regulations, the Director-General shall deliver certified copies thereof to the Secretary-General of the United Nations for registration in accordance with Article 102 of the Charter of the United Nations.

ANNEX 1

A. CORE CAPACITY REQUIREMENTS FOR SURVEILLANCE AND RESPONSE

1. States Parties shall utilize existing national structures and resources to meet their core capacity requirements under these Regulations, including with regard to:

(a) their surveillance, reporting, notification, verification, response and collaboration activities; and

(b) their activities concerning designated airports, ports and ground crossings.

2. Each State Party shall assess, within two years following the entry into force of these Regulations for that State Party, the ability of existing national structures and resources to meet the minimum requirements described in this Annex. As a result of such assessment, States Parties shall develop and implement plans of action to ensure that these core capacities are present and functioning throughout their territories as set out in paragraph 1 of Article 5 and paragraph 1 of Article 13.

3. States Parties and WHO shall support assessments, planning and implementation processes under this Annex.

4. At the local community level and/or primary public health response level

The capacities:

(a) to detect events involving disease or death above expected levels for the particular time and place in all areas within the territory of the State Party; and

(b) to report all available essential information immediately to the appropriate level of health-care response. At the community level, reporting shall be to local community health-care institutions or the appropriate health personnel. At the primary public health response level, reporting shall be to the intermediate or national response level, depending on organizational structures. For the purposes of this Annex, essential information includes the following: clinical descriptions, laboratory results, sources and type of risk, numbers of human cases and deaths, conditions affecting the spread of the disease and the health measures employed; and

(c) to implement preliminary control measures immediately.

5. At the intermediate public health response levels

The capacities:

(a) to confirm the status of reported events and to support or implement additional control measures; and

(b) to assess reported events immediately and, if found urgent, to report all essential information to the national level. For the purposes of this Annex, the criteria for urgent events include serious public health impact and/or unusual or unexpected nature with high potential for spread.

6. At the national level

Assessment and notification. The capacities:

(a) to assess all reports of urgent events within 48 hours; and

(b) to notify WHO immediately through the National IHR Focal Point when the assessment indicates the event is notifiable pursuant to paragraph 1 of Article 6 and Annex 2 and to inform WHO as required pursuant to Article 7 and paragraph 2 of Article 9.

Public health response. The capacities:

(a) to determine rapidly the control measures required to prevent domestic and international spread;

(b) to provide support through specialized staff, laboratory analysis of samples (domestically or through collaborating centres) and logistical assistance (e.g. equipment, supplies and transport);

(c) to provide on-site assistance as required to supplement local investigations;

(d) to provide a direct operational link with senior health and other officials to approve rapidly and implement containment and control measures;

(e) to provide direct liaison with other relevant government ministries;

(f) to provide, by the most efficient means of communication available, links with hospitals, clinics, airports, ports, ground crossings, laboratories and other key operational areas for the dissemination of information and recommendations received from WHO regarding events in the State Party's own territory and in the territories of other States Parties;

(g) to establish, operate and maintain a national public health emergency response plan, including the creation of multidisciplinary/multisectoral teams to respond to events that may constitute a public health emergency of international concern; and

(h) to provide the foregoing on a 24-hour basis.

B. CORE CAPACITY REQUIREMENTS FOR DESIGNATED AIRPORTS, PORTS AND GROUND CROSSINGS

1. At all times

The capacities:

(a) to provide access to (i) an appropriate medical service including diagnostic facilities located so as to allow the prompt assessment and care of ill travellers, and (ii) adequate staff, equipment and premises;

(b) to provide access to equipment and personnel for the transport of ill travellers to an appropriate medical facility;

(c) to provide trained personnel for the inspection of conveyances;

(d) to ensure a safe environment for travellers using point of entry facilities, including potable water supplies, eating establishments, flight catering facilities, public washrooms, appropriate solid and liquid waste disposal services and other potential risk areas, by conducting inspection programmes, as appropriate; and

(e) to provide as far as practicable a programme and trained personnel for the control of vectors and reservoirs in and near points of entry.

2. For responding to events that may constitute a public health emergency of international concern

The capacities:

(a) to provide appropriate public health emergency response by establishing and maintaining a public health emergency contingency plan, including the nomination of a coordinator and contact points for relevant point of entry, public health and other agencies and services;

(b) to provide assessment of and care for affected travellers or animals by establishing arrangements with local medical and veterinary facilities for their isolation, treatment and other support services that may be required;

(c) to provide appropriate space, separate from other travellers, to interview suspect or affected persons;

(d) to provide for the assessment and, if required, quarantine of suspect travellers, preferably in facilities away from the point of entry;

(e) to apply recommended measures to disinsect, derat, disinfect, decontaminate or otherwise treat baggage, cargo, containers, conveyances, goods or postal parcels including, when appropriate, at locations specially designated and equipped for this purpose;

(f) to apply entry or exit controls for arriving and departing travellers; and

(g) to provide access to specially designated equipment, and to trained personnel with appropriate personal protection, for the transfer of travellers who may carry infection or contamination.

ANNEX 2

DECISION INSTRUMENT FOR THE ASSESSMENT AND NOTIFICATION OF EVENTS THAT MAY CONSTITUTE A PUBLIC HEALTH EMERGENCY OF INTERNATIONAL CONCERN

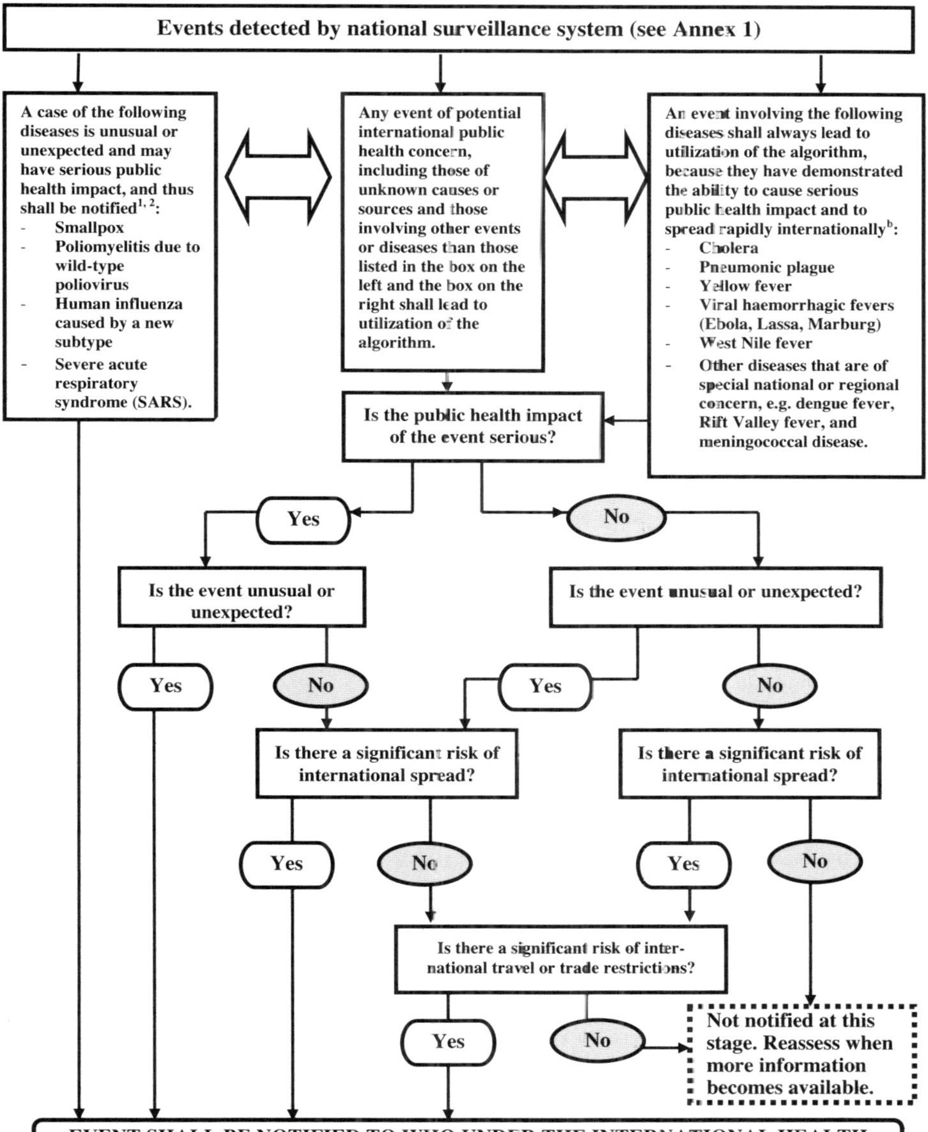

[1] As per WHO case definitions.

[2] The disease list shall be used only for the purposes of these Regulations.

EXAMPLES FOR THE APPLICATION OF THE DECISION INSTRUMENT FOR THE ASSESSMENT AND NOTIFICATION OF EVENTS THAT MAY CONSTITUTE A PUBLIC HEALTH EMERGENCY OF INTERNATIONAL CONCERN

The examples appearing in this Annex are not binding and are for indicative guidance purposes to assist in the interpretation of the decision instrument criteria.

DOES THE EVENT MEET AT LEAST TWO OF THE FOLLOWING CRITERIA?

<table>
<tr><td rowspan="5">Is the public health impact of the event serious?</td><td>I. Is the public health impact of the event serious?</td></tr>
<tr><td>1. Is the number of cases and/or number of deaths for this type of event large for the given place, time or population?</td></tr>
<tr><td>2. Has the event the potential to have a high public health impact?

THE FOLLOWING ARE EXAMPLES OF CIRCUMSTANCES THAT CONTRIBUTE TO HIGH PUBLIC HEALTH IMPACT:

✓ Event caused by a pathogen with high potential to cause epidemic (infectiousness of the agent, high case fatality, multiple transmission routes or healthy carrier).
✓ Indication of treatment failure (new or emerging antibiotic resistance, vaccine failure, antidote resistance or failure).
✓ Event represents a significant public health risk even if no or very few human cases have yet been identified.
✓ Cases reported among health staff.
✓ The population at risk is especially vulnerable (refugees, low level of immunization, children, elderly, low immunity, undernourished, etc.).
✓ Concomitant factors that may hinder or delay the public health response (natural catastrophes, armed conflicts, unfavourable weather conditions, multiple foci in the State Party).
✓ Event in an area with high population density.
✓ Spread of toxic, infectious or otherwise hazardous materials that may be occurring naturally or otherwise that has contaminated or has the potential to contaminate a population and/or a large geographical area.</td></tr>
<tr><td>3. Is external assistance needed to detect, investigate, respond and control the current event, or prevent new cases?

THE FOLLOWING ARE EXAMPLES OF WHEN ASSISTANCE MAY BE REQUIRED:

✓ Inadequate human, financial, material or technical resources – in particular:
– insufficient laboratory or epidemiological capacity to investigate the event (equipment, personnel, financial resources);
– insufficient antidotes, drugs and/or vaccine and/or protective equipment, decontamination equipment, or supportive equipment to cover estimated needs;
– existing surveillance system is inadequate to detect new cases in a timely manner.</td></tr>
<tr><td>IS THE PUBLIC HEALTH IMPACT OF THE EVENT SERIOUS?
Answer “yes” if you have answered “yes” to questions 1, 2 or 3 above.</td></tr>
</table>

Is the event unusual or unexpected?

II. Is the event unusual or unexpected?

4. *Is the event unusual?*

THE FOLLOWING ARE EXAMPLES OF UNUSUAL EVENTS:

- ✓ The event is caused by an unknown agent or the source, vehicle, route of transmission is unusual or unknown.
- ✓ Evolution of cases more severe than expected (including morbidity or case-fatality) or with unusual symptoms.
- ✓ Occurrence of the event itself unusual for the area, season or population.

5. *Is the event unexpected from a public health perspective?*

THE FOLLOWING ARE EXAMPLES OF UNEXPECTED EVENTS:

- ✓ Event caused by a disease/agent that had already been eliminated or eradicated from the State Party or not previously reported.

IS THE EVENT UNUSUAL OR UNEXPECTED?

Answer "yes" if you have answered "yes" to questions 4 or 5 above.

Is there a significant risk of international spread?

III. Is there a significant risk of international spread?

6. *Is there evidence of an epidemiological link to similar events in other States?*

7. *Is there any factor that should alert us to the potential for cross border movement of the agent, vehicle or host?*

THE FOLLOWING ARE EXAMPLES OF CIRCUMSTANCES THAT MAY PREDISPOSE TO INTERNATIONAL SPREAD:

- ✓ Where there is evidence of local spread, an index case (or other linked cases) with a history within the previous month of:
  - international travel (or time equivalent to the incubation period if the pathogen is known);
  - participation in an international gathering (pilgrimage, sports event, conference, etc.);
  - close contact with an international traveller or a highly mobile population.
- ✓ Event caused by an environmental contamination that has the potential to spread across international borders.
- ✓ Event in an area of intense international traffic with limited capacity for sanitary control or environmental detection or decontamination.

IS THERE A SIGNIFICANT RISK OF INTERNATIONAL SPREAD?

Answer "yes" if you have answered "yes" to questions 6 or 7 above.

<table>
<tr><td rowspan="6">Risk of international restrictions?</td><td>IV. Is there a significant risk of international travel or trade restrictions?</td></tr>
<tr><td>8. Have similar events in the past resulted in international restriction on trade and/or travel?</td></tr>
<tr><td>9. Is the source suspected or known to be a food product, water or any other goods that might be contaminated that has been exported/imported to/from other States?</td></tr>
<tr><td>10. Has the event occurred in association with an international gathering or in an area of intense international tourism?</td></tr>
<tr><td>11. Has the event caused requests for more information by foreign officials or international media?</td></tr>
<tr><td>IS THERE A SIGNIFICANT RISK OF INTERNATIONAL TRADE OR TRAVEL RESTRICTIONS?

Answer "yes" if you have answered "yes" to questions 8, 9, 10 or 11 above.</td></tr>
</table>

States Parties that answer "yes" to the question whether the event meets any two of the four criteria (I-IV) above, shall notify WHO under Article 6 of the International Health Regulations.

ANNEX 3

MODEL SHIP SANITATION CONTROL EXEMPTION CERTIFICATE/SHIP SANITATION CONTROL CERTIFICATE

Port of .... Date: ....

This Certificate records the inspection and 1) exemption from control or 2) control measures applied

Name of ship or inland navigation vessel ....Flag .... Registration/IMO No. ....

At the time of inspection the holds were unladen/laden with ...... tonnes of .... cargo

Name and address of inspecting officer ....

Ship Sanitation Control Exemption Certificate

Areas, [systems, and services] inspected	Evidence found[1]	Sample results[2]	Documents reviewed
Galley			Medical log
Pantry			Ship's log
Stores			Other
Hold(s)/cargo			
Quarters:			
- crew			
- officers			
- passengers			
- deck			
Potable water			
Sewage			
Ballast tanks			
Solid and medical waste			
Standing water			
Engine room			
Medical facilities			
Other areas specified - see attached			
Note areas not applicable, by marking N/A			

No evidence found. Ship/vessel is exempted from control measures.

Ship Sanitation Control Certificate

Control measures applied	Re-inspection date	Comments regarding conditions found

Control measures indicated were applied on the date below.

Name and designation of issuing officer .... Signature and seal .... Date ....

[1] (a) Evidence of infection or contamination, including: vectors in all stages of growth; animal reservoirs for vectors; rodents or other species that could carry human disease, microbiological, chemical and other risks to human health; signs of inadequate sanitary measures. (b) Information concerning any human cases (to be included in the Maritime Declaration of Health).

[2] Results from samples taken on board. Analysis to be provided to ship's master by most expedient means and, if re-inspection is required, to the next appropriate port of call coinciding with the re-inspection date specified in this certificate.

Sanitation Control Exemption Certificates and Sanitation Control Certificates are valid for a maximum of six months, but the validity period may be extended by one month if inspection cannot be carried out at the port and there is no evidence of infection or contamination.

ATTACHMENT TO MODEL SHIP SANITATION CONTROL EXEMPTION CERTIFICATE/SHIP SANITATION CONTROL CERTIFICATE

Areas/facilities/systems inspected[1]	Evidence found	Sample results	Documents reviewed	Control measures applied	Re-inspection date	Comments regarding conditions found
Food						
Source						
Storage						
Preparation						
Service						
Water						
Source						
Storage						
Distribution						
Waste						
Holding						
Treatment						
Disposal						
Swimming pools/spas						
Equipment						
Operation						
Medical facilities						
Equipment and medical devices						
Operation						
Medicines						
Other areas inspected						

[1] Indicate when the areas listed are not applicable by marking N/A.

ANNEX 4

TECHNICAL REQUIREMENTS PERTAINING TO CONVEYANCES AND CONVEYANCE OPERATORS

Section A Conveyance operators

1. Conveyance operators shall facilitate:

(a) inspections of the cargo, containers and conveyance;

(b) medical examinations of persons on board;

(c) application of other health measures under these Regulations; and

(d) provision of relevant public health information requested by the State Party.

2. Conveyance operators shall provide to the competent authority a valid Ship Sanitation Control Exemption Certificate or a Ship Sanitation Control Certificate or a Maritime Declaration of Health, or the Health Part of an Aircraft General Declaration, as required under these Regulations.

Section B Conveyances

1. Control measures applied to baggage, cargo, containers, conveyances and goods under these Regulations shall be carried out so as to avoid as far as possible injury or discomfort to persons or damage to the baggage, cargo, containers, conveyances and goods. Whenever possible and appropriate, control measures shall be applied when the conveyance and holds are empty.

2. States Parties shall indicate in writing the measures applied to cargo, containers or conveyances, the parts treated, the methods employed, and the reasons for their application. This information shall be provided in writing to the person in charge of an aircraft and, in case of a ship, on the Ship Sanitation Control Certificate. For other cargo, containers or conveyances, States Parties shall issue such information in writing to consignors, consignees, carriers, the person in charge of the conveyance or their respective agents.

ANNEX 5

SPECIFIC MEASURES FOR VECTOR-BORNE DISEASES

1. WHO shall publish, on a regular basis, a list of areas where disinsection or other vector control measures are recommended for conveyances arriving from these areas. Determination of such areas shall be made pursuant to the procedures regarding temporary or standing recommendations, as appropriate.

2. Every conveyance leaving a point of entry situated in an area where vector control is recommended should be disinsected and kept free of vectors. When there are methods and materials advised by the Organization for these procedures, these should be employed. The presence of vectors on board conveyances and the control measures used to eradicate them shall be included:

(a) in the case of aircraft, in the Health Part of the Aircraft General Declaration, unless this part of the Declaration is waived by the competent authority at the airport of arrival;

(b) in the case of ships, on the Ship Sanitation Control Certificates; and

(c) in the case of other conveyances, on a written proof of treatment issued to the consignor, consignee, carrier, the person in charge of the conveyance or their agent, respectively.

3. States Parties should accept disinsecting, deratting and other control measures for conveyances applied by other States if methods and materials advised by the Organization have been applied.

4. States Parties shall establish programmes to control vectors that may transport an infectious agent that constitutes a public health risk to a minimum distance of 400 metres from those areas of point of entry facilities that are used for operations involving travellers, conveyances, containers, cargo and postal parcels, with extension of the minimum distance if vectors with a greater range are present.

5. If a follow-up inspection is required to determine the success of the vector control measures applied, the competent authorities for the next known port or airport of call with a capacity to make such an inspection shall be informed of this requirement in advance by the competent authority advising such follow-up. In the case of ships, this shall be noted on the Ship Sanitation Control Certificate.

6. A conveyance may be regarded as suspect and should be inspected for vectors and reservoirs if:

(a) it has a possible case of vector-borne disease on board;

(b) a possible case of vector-borne disease has occurred on board during an international voyage; or

(c) it has left an affected area within a period of time where on-board vectors could still carry disease.

7. A State Party should not prohibit the landing of an aircraft or berthing of a ship in its territory if the control measures provided for in paragraph 3 of this Annex or otherwise recommended by the Organization are applied. However, aircraft or ships coming from an affected area may be required to land at airports or divert to another port specified by the State Party for that purpose.

8. A State Party may apply vector control measures to a conveyance arriving from an area affected by a vector-borne disease if the vectors for the foregoing disease are present in its territory.

ANNEX 6

VACCINATION, PROPHYLAXIS AND RELATED CERTIFICATES

1. Vaccines or other prophylaxis specified in Annex 7 or recommended under these Regulations shall be of suitable quality; those vaccines and prophylaxis designated by WHO shall be subject to its approval. Upon request, the State Party shall provide to WHO appropriate evidence of the suitability of vaccines and prophylaxis administered within its territory under these Regulations.

2. Persons undergoing vaccination or other prophylaxis under these Regulations shall be provided with an international certificate of vaccination or prophylaxis (hereinafter the "certificate") in the form specified in this Annex. No departure shall be made from the model of the certificate specified in this Annex.

3. Certificates under this Annex are valid only if the vaccine or prophylaxis used has been approved by WHO.

4. Certificates must be signed in the hand of the clinician, who shall be a medical practitioner or other authorized health worker, supervising the administration of the vaccine or prophylaxis. The certificate must also bear the official stamp of the administering centre; however, this shall not be an accepted substitute for the signature.

5. Certificates shall be fully completed in English or in French. They may also be completed in another language, in addition to either English or French.

6. Any amendment of this certificate, or erasure, or failure to complete any part of it, may render it invalid.

7. Certificates are individual and shall in no circumstances be used collectively. Separate certificates shall be issued for children.

8. A parent or guardian shall sign the certificate when the child is unable to write. The signature of an illiterate shall be indicated in the usual manner by the person's mark and the indication by another that this is the mark of the person concerned.

9. If the supervising clinician is of the opinion that the vaccination or prophylaxis is contraindicated on medical grounds, the supervising clinician shall provide the person with reasons, written in English or French, and where appropriate in another language in addition to English or French, underlying that opinion, which the competent authorities on arrival should take into account. The supervising clinician and competent authorities shall inform such persons of any risk associated with non-vaccination and with the non-use of prophylaxis in accordance with paragraph 4 of Article 23.

10. An equivalent document issued by the Armed Forces to an active member of those Forces shall be accepted in lieu of an international certificate in the form shown in this Annex if:

(a) it embodies medical information substantially the same as that required by such form; and

(b) it contains a statement in English or in French and where appropriate in another language in addition to English or French recording the nature and date of the vaccination or prophylaxis and to the effect that it is issued in accordance with this paragraph.

MODEL INTERNATIONAL CERTIFICATE OF VACCINATION OR PROPHYLAXIS

This is to certify that [name] ...., date of birth ...., sex ....,

nationality ...., national identification document, if applicable ....

whose signature follows ....

has on the date indicated been vaccinated or received prophylaxis against:

(name of disease or condition) ....

in accordance with the International Health Regulations.

Vaccine or prophylaxis	Date	Signature and professional status of supervising clinician	Manufacturer and batch No. of vaccine or prophylaxis	Certificate valid from .... until	Official stamp of administering centre
1.					
2.					

This certificate is valid only if the vaccine or prophylaxis used has been approved by the World Health Organization.

This certificate must be signed in the hand of the clinician, who shall be a medical practitioner or other authorized health worker, supervising the administration of the vaccine or prophylaxis. The certificate must also bear the official stamp of the administering centre; however, this shall not be an accepted substitute for the signature.

Any amendment of this certificate, or erasure, or failure to complete any part of it, may render it invalid.

The validity of this certificate shall extend until the date indicated for the particular vaccination or prophylaxis. The certificate shall be fully completed in English or in French. The certificate may also be completed in another language on the same document, in addition to either English or French.

ANNEX 7

REQUIREMENTS CONCERNING VACCINATION OR PROPHYLAXIS FOR SPECIFIC DISEASES

1. In addition to any recommendation concerning vaccination or prophylaxis, the following diseases are those specifically designated under these Regulations for which proof of vaccination or prophylaxis may be required for travellers as a condition of entry to a State Party:

Vaccination against yellow fever.

2. Recommendations and requirements for vaccination against yellow fever:

(a) For the purpose of this Annex:

(i) the incubation period of yellow fever is six days;

(ii) yellow fever vaccines approved by WHO provide protection against infection starting 10 days following the administration of the vaccine;

(iii) this protection continues for 10 years; and

(iv) the validity of a certificate of vaccination against yellow fever shall extend for a period of 10 years, beginning 10 days after the date of vaccination or, in the case of a revaccination within such period of 10 years, from the date of that revaccination.

(b) Vaccination against yellow fever may be required of any traveller leaving an area where the Organization has determined that a risk of yellow fever transmission is present.

(c) If a traveller is in possession of a certificate of vaccination against yellow fever which is not yet valid, the traveller may be permitted to depart, but the provisions of paragraph 2(h) of this Annex may be applied on arrival.

(d) A traveller in possession of a valid certificate of vaccination against yellow fever shall not be treated as suspect, even if coming from an area where the Organization has determined that a risk of yellow fever transmission is present.

(e) In accordance with paragraph 1 of Annex 6 the yellow fever vaccine used must be approved by the Organization.

(f) States Parties shall designate specific yellow fever vaccination centres within their territories in order to ensure the quality and safety of the procedures and materials employed.

(g) Every person employed at a point of entry in an area where the Organization has determined that a risk of yellow fever transmission is present, and every member of the crew of a conveyance using any such point of entry, shall be in possession of a valid certificate of vaccination against yellow fever.

(h) A State Party, in whose territory vectors of yellow fever are present, may require a traveller from an area where the Organization has determined that a risk of yellow fever transmission is present, who is unable to produce a valid certificate of vaccination against yellow fever, to be quarantined until the certificate becomes valid, or until a period of not more than six days, reckoned from the date of last possible exposure to infection, has elapsed, whichever occurs first.

(i) Travellers who possess an exemption from yellow fever vaccination, signed by an authorized medical officer or an authorized health worker, may nevertheless be allowed entry, subject to the provisions of the foregoing paragraph of this Annex and to being provided with information regarding protection from yellow fever vectors. Should the travellers not be quarantined, they may be required to report any feverish or other symptoms to the competent authority and be placed under surveillance.

ANNEX 8

MODEL OF MARITIME DECLARATION OF HEALTH

To be completed and submitted to the competent authorities by the masters of ships arriving from foreign ports.
Submitted at the port of .... Date ....
Name of ship or inland navigation vessel .... Registration/IMO No ....arriving from ....sailing to ....
(Nationality)(Flag of vessel) .... Master's name ....
Gross tonnage (ship) ....
Tonnage (inland navigation vessel) ....
Valid Sanitation Control Exemption/Control Certificate carried on board? Yes .... No .... Issued at .... date ....
Re-inspection required? Yes .... No ....
Has ship/vessel visited an affected area identified by the World Health Organization? Yes ..... No .....
Port and date of visit ....
List ports of call from commencement of voyage with dates of departure, or within past thirty days, whichever is shorter:
....

Upon request of the competent authority at the port of arrival, list crew members, passengers or other persons who have joined ship/vessel since international voyage began or within past thirty days, whichever is shorter, including all ports/countries visited in this period (add additional names to the attached schedule):

(1) Name ....joined from: (1) ....(2) ....(3) ....
(2) Name ....joined from: (1) ....(2) ....(3) ....
(3) Name ....joined from: (1) ....(2) ....(3) ....

Number of crew members on board ....
Number of passengers on board ....

Health questions

(1) Has any person died on board during the voyage otherwise than as a result of accident? Yes .... No .....
If yes, state particulars in attached schedule. Total no. of deaths ....

(2) Is there on board or has there been during the international voyage any case of disease which you suspect to be of an infectious nature? Yes........ No........ If yes, state particulars in attached schedule.

(3) Has the total number of ill passengers during the voyage been greater than normal/expected? Yes .... No .....
How many ill persons? ....

(4) Is there any ill person on board now? Yes .... No .... If yes, state particulars in attached schedule.

(5) Was a medical practitioner consulted? Yes .... No ...... If yes, state particulars of medical treatment or advice provided in attached schedule.

(6) Are you aware of any condition on board which may lead to infection or spread of disease? Yes .... No ....
If yes, state particulars in attached schedule.

(7) Has any sanitary measure (e.g. quarantine, isolation, disinfection or decontamination) been applied on board? Yes .... No ......
If yes, specify type, place and date ....

(8) Have any stowaways been found on board? Yes .... No ...... If yes, where did they join the ship (if known)? ....

(9) Is there a sick animal or pet on board? Yes .... No ....

Note: In the absence of a surgeon, the master should regard the following symptoms as grounds for suspecting the existence of a disease of an infectious nature:

(a) fever, persisting for several days or accompanied by (i) prostration; (ii) decreased consciousness; (iii) glandular swelling; (iv) jaundice; (v) cough or shortness of breath; (vi) unusual bleeding; or (vii) paralysis.

(b) with or without fever: (i) any acute skin rash or eruption; (ii) severe vomiting (other than sea sickness); (iii) severe diarrhoea; or (iv) recurrent convulsions.

I hereby declare that the particulars and answers to the questions given in this Declaration of Health (including the schedule) are true and correct to the best of my knowledge and belief.

Signed ....

Master

Countersigned ....

Ship's Surgeon (if carried)

Date ....

ATTACHMENT TO MODEL OF MARITIME DECLARATION OF HEALTH

Name	Class or rating	Age	Sex	Nationality	Port, date joined ship/vessel	Nature of illness	Date of onset of symptoms	Reported to a port medical officer?	Disposal of case[1]	Drugs, medicines or other treatment given to patient	Comments

[1] State: (1) whether the person recovered, is still ill or died; and (2) whether the person is still on board, was evacuated (including the name of the port or airport), or was buried at sea.

ANNEX 9

THIS DOCUMENT IS PART OF THE AIRCRAFT GENERAL DECLARATION, PROMULGATED BY THE INTERNATIONAL CIVIL AVIATION ORGANIZATION

HEALTH PART OF THE AIRCRAFT GENERAL DECLARATION[1]

Declaration of Health

Name and seat number or function of persons on board with illnesses other than airsickness or the effects of accidents, who may be suffering from a communicable disease (a fever - temperature 38°C/100 °F or greater - associated with one or more of the following signs or symptoms, e.g. appearing obviously unwell; persistent coughing; impaired breathing; persistent diarrhoea; persistent vomiting; skin rash; bruising or bleeding without previous injury; or confusion of recent onset, increases the likelihood that the person is suffering a communicable disease) as well as such cases of illness disembarked during a previous stop ....

....

Details of each disinsecting or sanitary treatment (place, date, time, method) during the flight. If no disinsecting has been carried out during the flight, give details of most recent disinsecting

....

....

Signature, if required, with time and date ____

Crew member concerned

[1] This version of the Aircraft General Declaration entered into force on 15 July 2007. The full document may be obtained from the website of the International Civil Aviation Organization at http://www.icao.int.

APPENDIX 1

STATES PARTIES TO THE INTERNATIONAL HEALTH REGULATIONS (2005) [1]

Except as otherwise indicated, the International Health Regulations (2005) entered into force on 15 June 2007 for the following States:

Afghanistan, Albania, Algeria, Andorra, Angola, Antigua and Barbuda, Argentina, Armenia, Australia, Austria, Azerbaijan, Bahamas, Bahrain, Bangladesh, Barbados, Belarus, Belgium, Belize, Benin, Bhutan, Bolivia, Bosnia and Herzegovina, Botswana, Brazil, Brunei Darussalam, Bulgaria, Burkina Faso, Burundi, Cambodia, Cameroon, Canada, Cape Verde, Central African Republic, Chad, Chile, China[2], Colombia, Comoros, Congo, Cook Islands, Costa Rica, Côte d'Ivoire, Croatia, Cuba, Cyprus, Czech Republic, Democratic People's Republic of Korea, Democratic Republic of the Congo, Denmark, Djibouti, Dominica, Dominican Republic, Ecuador, Egypt, El Salvador, Equatorial Guinea, Eritrea, Estonia, Ethiopia, Fiji, Finland, France, Gabon, Gambia, Georgia, Germany, Ghana, Greece[2], Grenada, Guatemala, Guinea, Guinea-Bissau, Guyana, Haiti, Holy See, Honduras, Hungary, Iceland, India (8 August 2007)[2], Indonesia, Iran (Islamic Republic of)[2], Iraq, Ireland, Israel, Italy, Jamaica, Japan, Jordan, Kazakhstan, Kenya, Kiribati, Kuwait, Kyrgyzstan, Lao People's Democratic Republic, Latvia, Lebanon, Lesotho, Liberia, Libyan Arab Jamahiriya, Lithuania, Luxembourg, Madagascar, Malawi, Malaysia, Maldives, Mali, Malta, Marshall Islands, Mauritania, Mauritius, Mexico, Micronesia (Federated States of), Monaco, Mongolia, Montenegro (5 February 2008), Morocco, Mozambique, Myanmar, Namibia, Nauru, Nepal, Netherlands, New Zealand, Nicaragua, Niger, Nigeria, Niue, Norway, Oman, Pakistan, Palau, Panama, Papua New Guinea, Paraguay, Peru, Philippines, Poland, Portugal[2], Qatar, Republic of Korea, Moldova, Romania, Russian Federation, Rwanda, Saint Kitts and Nevis, Saint Lucia, Saint Vincent and the Grenadines, Samoa, San Marino, Sao Tome and Principe, Saudi Arabia, Senegal, Serbia, Seychelles, Sierra Leone, Singapore, Slovakia, Slovenia, Solomon Islands, Somalia, South Africa, Spain, Sri Lanka, Sudan, Suriname, Swaziland, Sweden, Switzerland, Syrian Arab Republic, Tajikistan, Thailand, The former Yugoslav Republic of Macedonia, Timor-Leste, Togo, Tonga[2], Trinidad and Tobago, Tunisia, Turkey[2], Turkmenistan, Tuvalu, Uganda, Ukraine, United Arab Emirates, United Kingdom of Great Britain and Northern Ireland, United Republic of Tanzania, United States of America (18 July 2007) [2], Uruguay, Uzbekistan, Vanuatu, Venezuela (Bolivarian Republic of), Viet Nam, Yemen, Zambia, Zimbabwe.

---

[1] At 5 February 2008.

[2] Indicates that a State Party has submitted, to the Director-General of WHO, documentation related to the International Health Regulations (2005), which has been circulated by the Director-General to all Member States of WHO as well as to other States eligible to become Parties to the Regulations pursuant to Article 64 thereof.

APPENDIX 2

RESERVATIONS AND OTHER STATE PARTY COMMUNICATIONS IN CONNECTION WITH THE INTERNATIONAL HEALTH REGULATIONS (2005) [1, 2]

I. RESERVATIONS AND UNDERSTANDINGS

INDIA

I am directed to refer to Reservations in respect of India mentioned in Annexure-II to IHR 1969 (Revised upto 1983) {copy enclosed} and to request you to notify the following Reservations in respect of India for notification under Article 62 of the recently circulated IHR 2005 :-

Proposed Reservation to IHR 2005:-

1. The Government of India reserves the right to consider the whole territory of a country as infected with yellow fever whenever yellow fever has been notified under Article 6 and other relevant articles in this regard of IHR (2005). The Government of India reserves the right to continue to regard an area as infected with yellow fever until there is definite evidence that yellow-fever infection has been completely eradicated from that area.
2. Yellow Fever disease will be treated as disease of Public health emergency of international concern and all health measures being applied presently like disinsection of conveyance, vaccination requirements and quarantine of passengers and crew (as may be required) (as per Article 7, 9.2(b), 42 and relevant annexures) will be continued as has been stipulated under Annex-II of IHR-1969 (Revised in 1983).

UNITED STATES OF AMERICA

The Mission, by means of this note, informs the Acting Director-General of the World Health Organization that the Government of the United States of America accepts the IHRs, subject to the reservation and understandings referred to below.

The Mission, by means of this note, and in accordance with Article 22 of the Constitution of the World Health Organization and Article 59(1) of the IHRs, submits the following reservation on behalf of the Government of the United States of America:

The Government of the United States of America reserves the right to assume obligations under these Regulations in a manner consistent with its fundamental principles of federalism. With respect to obligations concerning the development, strengthening, and maintenance of the core capacity requirements set forth in Annex 1, these Regulations shall be implemented by the Federal Government

---

[1] At 5 February 2008.

[2] This Appendix reproduces the relevant parts of the communications submitted by States, which have been edited by the Secretariat of WHO, or translations thereof. Copies of the original communications are available at http://www.who.int/ihr.

or the state governments, as appropriate and in accordance with our Constitution, to the extent that the implementation of these obligations comes under the legal jurisdiction of the Federal Government. To the extent that such obligations come under the legal jurisdiction of the state governments, the Federal Government shall bring such obligations with a favorable recommendation to the notice of the appropriate state authorities.

The Mission, by means of this note, also submits three understandings on behalf of the Government of the United States of America. The first understanding relates to the application of the IHRs to incidents involving natural, accidental or deliberate release of chemical, biological or radiological materials:

In view of the definitions of "disease," "event," and "public health emergency of international concern" as set forth in Article 1 of these Regulations, the notification requirements of Articles 6 and 7, and the decision instrument and guidelines set forth in Annex 2, the United States understands that States Parties to these Regulations have assumed an obligation to notify to WHO potential public health emergencies of international concern, irrespective of origin or source, whether they involve the natural, accidental or deliberate release of biological, chemical or radionuclear materials.

The second understanding relates to the application of Article 9 of the IHRs:

Article 9 of these Regulations obligates a State Party "as far as practicable" to notify the World Health Organization (WHO) of evidence received by that State of a public health risk occurring outside of its territory that may result in the international spread of disease. Among other notifications that could prove to be impractical under this article, it is the United States' understanding that any notification that would undermine the ability of the U.S. Armed Forces to operate effectively in pursuit of U.S. national security interests would not be considered practical for purposes of this Article.

The third understanding relates to the question of whether the IHRs create judicially enforceable private rights. Based on its delegation's participation in the negotiations of the IHRs, the Government of the United States of America does not believe that the IHRs were intended to create judicially enforceable private rights:

The United States understands that the provisions of the Regulations do not create judicially enforceable private rights.

II. OBJECTIONS TO RESERVATIONS AND UNDERSTANDINGS

IRAN (Islamic Republic of)

The Permanent Mission of the Islamic Republic of Iran to the United Nations Office and other International Organizations in Geneva presents its compliments to the World Health Organization and with reference to note verbale No. C.L.2.2007 dated 17 January 2007 concerning the Reservation and Understandings of the Government of the United States of America on the International Health Regulations (IHR), has the honor to convey the official objection of the Government of the Islamic Republic of Iran to the same Reservation and Understandings, based on the following:

According to the IHR, while "States may make reservations to these Regulations", "such reservations shall not be incompatible with the object and purpose of these regulations". Furthermore, in accordance with the IHR, "the implementation of these Regulations shall be guided by the goal of their universal application for the protection of all people of the world from the international spread of disease".

The Government of the Islamic Republic of Iran believes that, by giving more prominence to federalism than its obligations under the IHR, the reserving Government attempts to evade its due responsibilities and obligations. The aforementioned Government, by adopting a selective approach, provides its states with the option of exempting themselves from full compliance with the provisions of the IHR. Since implementation of the IHR largely depends on the development, strengthening and maintenance of the core capacity requirements set forth in Annex 1, reservation of such a general nature leads to undermining the IHR foundations as well as its integrity and universal applicability. Such reservation is considered to be incompatible with the object and purpose of these Regulations and is, therefore, unacceptable.

Moreover, the understandings and interpretations assumed by a government, too, should not affect the obligations to be undertaken by that government and must not be incompatible with the object and purpose of the Regulations.

As regards to the first Understanding of the reserving Government, it must be recalled that the majority of W.H.O. Member States participating in the IHR negotiations, categorically rejected the inclusion of the related interpretation within the provisions of the IHR. Their rejections were prompted to avoid confusion over respective obligations of the State Parties under the IHR and to preempt overlapping of the competencies and duplication of work among the relevant intergovernmental organizations or international bodies. Article 6.1 and 14.2 of the IHR address such concerns.

The second Understanding attempts to dilute the obligations of the U.S. Government under the IHR. It is an attempt to place national interests above the treaty obligations by excluding the U.S. Armed Forces from the IHR bindings. The universal applicability of the IHR for the protection of all peoples of the world from the international spread of diseases leaves no room for exempting the American Armed Forces, in particular those operating abroad. Such an exemption could not be conceded to, taking into account the nature, direction and possible public health consequences of the U.S. Armed Forces operations. It should be recalled that during IHR negotiations, the majority of W.H.O. Member States strongly rejected the above exclusion proposed by the U.S. Government. It is, therefore, in violation of the U.S. obligations under the IHR and is incompatible with the object and purpose of these regulations, to which the Government of the Islamic Republic of Iran strongly objects.

The Government of the Islamic Republic of Iran reiterates that it does not consider the Reservation and the two Understandings stated by the U.S. Government, as legally binding.

III. DECLARATIONS AND STATEMENTS

CHINA[1]

1. The Government of the People's Republic of China decides that the *International Health Regulations (2005)* (hereinafter referred to as "the IHR") applies to the entire territory of the People's Republic of China, including the Hong Kong Special Administrative Region, the Macau Special Administrative Region and the Taiwan Province.

2. The Ministry of Health of the People's Republic of China is designated as China's National Focal Point, pursuant to Paragraph 1 of Article 4 of the IHR. The local health administrative authorities are the health authorities responsible for the implementation of the IHR in their respective

[1] English translation provided by the Government.

jurisdictions. The General Administration of Quality Supervision, Inspection and Quarantine of the People's Republic of China and its local offices are the competent authorities of the points of entry referred to in Article 22 of the IHR.

3. To meet the needs of applying the IHR, the Government of the People's Republic of China is revising the *Frontier Health and Quarantine Law of the People's Republic of China.* It has incorporated the development, enhancement and maintenance of the core capability-building for rapid and effective response to public health hazards and public health emergencies of international concern into its program of establishing a national health emergency response system during the 11th Five-year Plan for National Economic and Social Development. It is formulating the technical standards for the surveillance, reporting, assessment, determination and notification of public health emergencies of international concern. It has established an inter-agency information-sharing and coordination mechanism for implementing the IHR. And it has conducted cooperation and exchanges with relevant states parties on the implementation of the IHR.

4. The Government of the People's Republic of China endorses and will implement the resolution of the 59th World Health Assembly calling upon its member states to comply immediately, on a voluntary basis, with provisions of the IHR considered relevant to the risk posed by the avian influenza and pandemic influenza.

GREECE

Reply dated 24 January 2007 to the statement made by the Republic of Turkey on 14 December 2006

The Permanent Mission of Greece to the United Nations Office and other International Organizations in Geneva presents its compliments to the Director General of the World Health Organization and, with reference to the latter's Note Verbale under ref.no. C.L.3.2007, dated January 17th, 2007, and the Note Verbale enclosed therein of the Permanent Mission of the Republic of Turkey ref. no 520.20/2006/BMCO DT/12201, dated December 14th, 2006, has the honour to draw the attention of the Director General to the fact that the correct title of the Montreux Convention regarding the regime of the straights of the Dardanelles, the Marmara sea and the Bosporus is: "The Convention Regarding the Regime of the Straights signed at Montreux on July 20th, 1936".

Furthermore, concerning the reference made in the aforementioned Note Verbale of the Permanent Mission of Turkey to the maritime traffic regulations unilaterally adopted in Turkey in 1998, we would like to remind the Director General that they are in contravention to the provisions of the International Law of the Sea, the Montreux Convention and the relevant rules and Recommendations of the International Maritime Organization adopted on June 1st, 1994.

Reply dated 16 April 2007 to the Note Verbale from the Permanent Mission of Turkey dated 1 March 2007

A. Firstly, it should be noted that there is no substantive link between the content of the Turkish statement contained in Note Verbale 520.20/BMCO DT/12201 dated 14th December 2006 and the new International Health Regulations. In fact, the Turkish statement seeks to elicit tacit acceptance or recognition of the national regulations, adopted by Turkey, concerning maritime traffic through the Straits.

However, these regulations were adopted unilaterally and were not approved by the International Maritime Organization or the parties of the Montreux Convention of 1936 which governs the issue.

Concerning its precise content, the statement goes on to assert that Turkey rightly points out that as far as the implementation of the new International Health Regulations for maritime traffic in the Straits is concerned, this should be done in accordance with the provisions of the Montreux Convention of 1936 regarding the regime of the Straits. It is, however, self-evident that the new Health Regulations do not influence the existing international regime of navigation through the Straits, neither could they do so, as there is no connection of substance between them.

The Turkish statement goes on to assert that the Turkish Maritime Traffic Regulations of 1998 will also be taken into account. This means that the Turkish Authorities will enforce the International Health Regulations subject to certain ill-defined national modifications, which are in fact themselves in contravention of the international obligations Turkey has undertaken under the Montreux Convention.

Furthermore, the Turkish Authorities reserve the right to also take into account any further revision of their national traffic regulations, to be adopted in the same unilateral way in the future. In fact, this would seem simply that, in so far as the Straits are concerned, Turkey may implement the new International Heath Regulations as it sees fit.

The reference, therefore, to national legislation and to any future revisions of this legislation, while irrelevant to the subject at hand, is nonetheless problematic because it seeks to subject international conventional obligations to national rules and regulations.

B. Furthermore, the Turkish Regulations concerning traffic in the Straits are themselves not in conformity with:

- The 1936 Montreux Convention: this Convention enshrines full freedom of navigation (articles 1 and 2) through the Straits without any restrictions whatsoever (apart from sanitary control) and without any formalities, irrespective of the kind of cargo or the timing of the transit. Thus, the Turkish Regulations by, amongst other things, imposing a compulsory reporting system (Reg. 6, 25 and al.) and, particularly, by providing for the possibility of the total suspension of traffic (Reg.20) are incompatible with the Montreux Convention.

- The IMO Rules and Regulations: Paragraphs 1.2 and 1.3 foresee that only in the case where a vessel is unable to comply with the Traffic Separation Scheme do the Turkish Authorities have the right to temporarily suspend two-way traffic and to regulate the resulting one way traffic. The IMO Rules and Regulations on no account foresee a total suspension of traffic in the Straits. The Turkish Regulations, on the other hand, provide for the possibility to completely suspend traffic in general for a wide variety of reasons.

- The international law of the sea regarding navigation through international straits: such law encourages cooperation in order to ensure the safe transit of vessels through the Straits and in order to protect the environment. The Turkish Regulations, however, were adopted unilaterally, in contravention of the law of the sea and the relevant law of treaties.

C. As to the Turkish Note dated 1st March 2007 (Ref. No: 520.20/2007/BMCO DT/1711), the information contained there in is inaccurate on several points. More specifically, the said Turkish Note states:

- that the Turkish Regulations "have been put into effect taking into account Turkey's obligations and rights arising from the Montreux Convention", whereas the latter contains and rights arising from the Montreux Convention", whereas the latter contains no provision which authorizes Turkey to unilaterally issue traffic regulations.

- that Turkey "informed IMO of the safety measures taken in the Straits", whereas Turkey has consistently refused to officially submit its national regulations to IMO for discussion and examination, alleging that it is a matter of exclusive Turkish jurisdiction.

- that "...Traffic Separation Schemes and Reporting System... were adopted by IMO together with some other rules in 1995", whereas only Traffic Separation Schemes were adopted by that Organization, together with the relevant IMO Rules and Recommendations. The Reporting System included in the Turkish Regulations was never adopted by IMO.

- that "...the maritime Safety Committee of the IMO confirmed at its 71st session that the routing system and the associated IMO Rules and Recommendations... had contributed significantly to an increase in safety ..." in an attempt to create the impression that the IMO is referring to the Turkish Regulations, whereas it is only referring to the measures adopted within the IMO itself.

In the light of the above, Greece considers the statement made by Turkey in its Note Verbale 520.20/2006/BMCO DT/12201 dated 14th December 2006 as irrelevant to the International Health Regulations, thus having no legal effect as to the latter's implementation. Furthermore, Greece reiterates the point made in her Note Verbale no. (331) 6395/5/AS 168 dated 24 January 2007 as to the importance of using the correct terminology when referring to international instruments such as the Montreux Convention.

PORTUGAL

Declaration of the Presidency of the Council of the European Union (EU) on the reservation of the Government of the United States of America concerning the International Health Regulations

The International Health Regulations (IHR) are a very effective tool for reinforcing the connection between the surveillance systems and in establishing rapid reaction mechanisms. The EC and its 27 Member States have strongly supported the revised IHR, which recently came into force, and we will continue this support for the implementation of the IHR in full and without restrictions.

The EC and its 27 Member States take note of the above mentioned reservation and declare that they understand it to mean that, in accordance with the principle that a Party may not invoke the provisions of its internal law as justification for its failure to perform its international obligations, this reservation in no way intends to question the obligations stemming from the IHR. The EC and its 27 Member States understand that the Federal Government of the United States of America fully recognises those obligations and that it will exercise every effort to ensure that the provisions of the IHR are fully implemented and given full effect by the pertinent authorities in the United States of America.

Declaration of the Presidency of the Council of the European Union (EU) on the statement of the Government of Turkey concerning the International Health Regulations

The International Health Regulations (IHR) are a very effective tool for reinforcing the connection between the surveillance systems and in establishing rapid reaction mechanisms. The EC and its 27 Member States have strongly supported the revised IHR, which recently came into force, and we will continue this support for the implementation of the IHR in full and without restrictions.

The EC and its 27 Member States take note of Turkey's intention to implement the provisions of the IHR in accordance with the Convention regarding the regime of the Straits, signed at Montreux on 20 July 1936.

The EC and its 27 Member States understand the desire of the Turkish authorities to respect their international obligations, such as the Montreux Convention regarding traffic in the Straits. In this respect they would like to refer to Article 57 of the IHR, which provides that States parties recognize that the IHR and other relevant international agreements should be interpreted so as to be compatible. The provisions of the IHR shall not affect the rights and obligations of any State party deriving from other international agreements.

Concerning the reference by Turkey to internal legislation which has no direct bearing on the implementation of the IHR, the EC and its 27 Member States understand that Turkey will ensure that the application of its internal legislation fully respects the letter and spirit of the IHR and the regime of freedom of navigation in the Straits as established by the Montreux Convention.

Declaration of the Presidency of the Council of the European Union (EU) on the reservation of the Government of India concerning the International Health Regulations

The International Health Regulations (IHR) are a very effective tool for reinforcing the connection between the surveillance systems and in establishing rapid reaction mechanisms. The EC and its 27 Member States have strongly supported the revised IHR, which recently came into force, and we will continue this support for the implementation of the IHR in full and without restrictions.

The EC and its 27 Member States understand the willingness of the Government of India to apply strong measures in order to keep the territory of India free of yellow fever. The EC and its 27 Member States recognise the challenges in ensuring the surveillance and protection of such a large territory, considering the existence of factors (e.g. presence of aedes) which may facilitate the spread of contamination.

The EC and its 27 Member States nevertheless expect that this reservation will be implemented in a reasonable way, considering the potentially unnecessary interference it could have with international traffic and trade from the largest part of the geographical territory of the EC in the case of a yellow fever outbreak in an outermost region of the EU or in a non-European part of a Member State of the EC (e.g. Guyana, Antilles). The fact that the Government of India considers yellow fever to be a notifiable disease should not trigger disproportionate control measures.

The commitment of the EC and its 27 Member States to ensure the rapid and comprehensive implementation of the IHR will reinforce the measures already implemented to maintain the whole territory of the EC free of yellow fever.

TURKEY

Statement made by the Republic of Turkey on 14 December 2006

Turkey will implement the provisions of the International Health Regulations in accordance with the Convention regarding the regime of the Turkish Straits, signed at Montreux on 20 July 1936, as well as by taking into account Turkish 1998 Maritime Traffic Regulations for the Turkish Straits and any future revisions to be made thereto.

Reply dated 1 March 2007 to the Note Verbale from the Permanent Mission of Greece dated 24 January 2007

The Maritime Traffic Regulations for the Turkish Straits have been put into effect taking into account Turkey's obligations and rights arising from the Montreux Convention. The said Regulations do not contain any element that is in contravention of international law or International Maritime Organization's (IMO) Rules and Recommendations and are being implemented accordingly.

The measures taken in the Turkish Straits in accordance with the said Regulations are aimed at improving the safety of navigation, human life, cultural and environmental heritage. Moreover, the safety measures are needed vis-à-vis the risks and dangers of passage of the increased number of tanker traffic in the Straits.

Turkey has duly informed IMO of the safety measures taken in the Straits. Besides, Traffic Separation Schemes and Reporting System, established within the framework of the Turkish Straits Regulations, were adopted by IMO together with some other rules in 1995.

Furthermore, the Maritime Safety Committee of the IMO confirmed at its 71st session on May 1999 that the routeing system and the associated IMO Rules and Recommendations relating to the Turkish Straits have proven to be effective and successful and had contributed significantly to an increase in safety and a reduction of the risk of collisions.

The Turkish Straits Vessel Traffic Services which have been functioning since 31 December 2003 within the framework of the Montreux Convention, IMO Rules and the Turkish Straits Regulations, provide traffic arrangements successfully with high standard technical equipment and qualified expert personnel.

Accordingly, the arguments in the above-mentioned Note of the Permanent Mission of Greece are unfounded and the statement of Turkey registered in our Note dated 14 December 2006 (Ref. no: 520.20/2006/BMCO DT/12201) remains unchanged and valid.

IV. DECLARATIONS UNDER ARTICLE 59, PARAGRAPH 3, OF THE IHR (2005)

TONGA

Following their adoption by the World Health Assembly in May 2005, the International Health Regulations (IHR) 2005 will enter into force on 15 June 2007.

The Kingdom of Tonga supports the important contribution the IHR 2005 will make to the strengthening of national and global systems for the protection of public health from the spread of disease.

The Kingdom of Tonga understands that in order to be effective, the IHR 2005 will need to operate at various levels within each country, as well as between countries internationally and the World Health Organization. With this in mind, Tonga has, with support from regional partners including WHO, taken a number of steps to prepare for the entry into force of the new regime. However, it is not possible to confirm that all the required adjustments will be able to be achieved by 15 June 2007.

Therefore, on behalf of the Kingdom of Tonga, and in accordance with paragraph 3 of Article 59 of the IHR 2005, I declare that the following adjustments may not be completed by June 2007.

The outstanding adjustments are as follows:

1. Complete the review of the Public Health Act 1992 to ensure legislative consistency with the IHR 2005;

2. Strengthen existing systems for the regular, national reporting of notifiable diseases, including the reporting of any events of potential public health significance, irrespective of their source;

3. Various enhancements to border health protection functions, including improved reporting and response capacities for public health events at Fua'amotu Airport and surveillance and control of vector/reservoir species at Fua'amotu airport and the seaport at Nuku'alofa.

The Kingdom of Tonga is, and will remain, committed to playing its part in the collective actions that contribute to the protection of public health for all people of the world. It is my intention that the outstanding adjustments will be achieved by 31 December 2007, and certainly no later than 15 June 2008.

INDEX TO THE INTERNATIONAL HEALTH REGULATIONS

The figures refer to page numbers and not to articles of the Regulations as was the case in the first edition.

H

I

Q

R

S